SWITCH ON
YOUR BRAIN
Every Day

365 READINGS for PEAK HAPPINESS, THINKING, and HEALTH

DR. CAROLINE LEAF

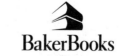

BakerBooks
a division of Baker Publishing Group
Grand Rapids, Michigan

© 2018 by Caroline Leaf

Published by Baker Books
a division of Baker Publishing Group
PO Box 6287, Grand Rapids, MI 49516-6287
www.bakerbooks.com

Printed in the United States of America

Library of Congress Cataloging-in-Publication Control Number: 2018014309

ISBN: 978-0-8010-9360-9

Old Testament Scripture quotations are taken from the New Revised Standard Version of the Bible, copyright © 1989, by the Division of Christian Education of the National Council of the Churches of Christ in the United States of America. Used by permission. All rights reserved.

New Testament Scripture quotations are taken from *The Kingdom New Testament* by N. T. Wright (New York: HarperOne, 2011). Copyright © 2011 by Nicholas Thomas Wright. Used by permission.

18 19 20 21 22 23 24   7 6 5 4 3 2 1

In keeping with biblical principles of creation stewardship, Baker Publishing Group advocates the responsible use of our natural resources. As a member of the Green Press Initiative, our company uses recycled paper when possible. The text paper of this book is composed in part of post-consumer waste.

green press INITIATIVE

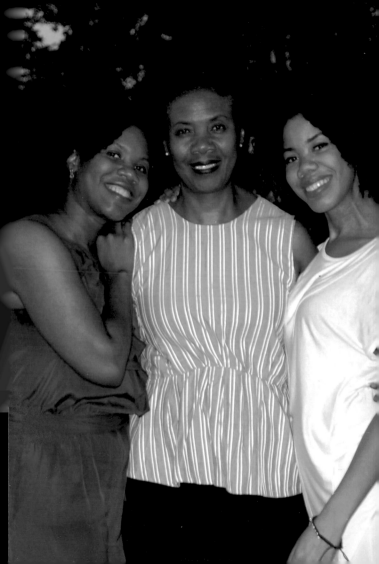

Introduction

How to Get the Most out of These Readings

The Bible truly is a remarkable set of books. It contains so much: so many narratives, so many characters, so many emotions, so many events, so many eras.[1] It is shaped, stretched, and colored by the hopes, dreams, fears, and choices of the past, present, and future. It is the story of human effort, human victory, and, of course, human failure. It reverberates with the need for a transcendent purpose, a life greater than the sum of its parts.[2] And, after thousands of years, we have barely scratched its surface. After thousands of reads, we still have so much more to see and understand. It is not merely a series of documents set in the stone of time; it is a book of books that has a life of its own: it is in many ways "the living Word."

The Bible is rather like the human mind. Dynamic, brilliant, powerful, and influential, it cannot be used with abandon, as it impacts not only the reader but the world. It is intricate and both obscure and transparent. It cannot be divorced from the context of human experience. Jesus came to earth as a man: the incarnated God firmly planted himself in the midst of human history, with all its intrigues, variations, and undertakings. Human community, after all, preceded the written word.[3] The Bible is therefore a collection of narratives that both reflects and shapes our memories and thus our identity, just as our thoughts shape what we think, say, and do.

With the advent of quantum physics, I would even go as far as to say that mind, or consciousness, underscores the biblical narrative from Genesis to Revelation. "In the beginning was the Word . . ." Perhaps one of the most iconic verses in the Bible, John 1:1, hearkens back to Genesis in a dramatic fashion, highlighting the significance of the Word, the *logos*, which in the Greek means reason, intellect, or intelligibility.[4] This reason, this divine intelligence, shapes our existence, reworking the lines and sketches of our daily life. *Logos*, the divine consciousness,[5] brings order to chaos, peace to destruction, love to hatred. God was, is, and always will be. He upholds the universe.

As I discussed in *Switch On Your Brain*, quantum physics helps us understand the importance of consciousness, or *logos*, in the Bible. Quantum physics, with its examination of science beyond the traditional paradigms of space and time, points directly to the belief that the universe has a creative mind behind it (consciousness) and therefore a creative purpose. Elementary particles like atoms and electrons are not "things" per se.[6] These particles form a world of pure possibilities, which are made into actualities through the choices of the observer.[7] We essentially create realities with our minds. And God is the ultimate reality. He is always observing, always present. Through him all things have their existence. Through him all things are made, and made new (Gen. 1–2; 2 Cor. 5:17). If God is love, then love underpins the universe (1 John 4:8). Essentially, perfect love is the raison d'être for every "thing" as a thing that exists.

But what does all this have to do with us? If we are created in the image of God (Gen. 1:27), if we have the mind of the Messiah (1 Cor. 2:16), if we are the children of God (Gal. 3:26), if we are called to reflect his glory (2 Cor. 3:18), and if we are the high priests and stewards of creation (Gen. 2:15), we have this power: the power of mind. Now that is certainly something to get excited about! It is also something we ought to take very seriously. We cannot call ourselves sons or daughters of the Most High God without realizing that our thoughts, feelings, and choices impact not only us but everyone and everything around us. We create realities that transform our world. It is up to us to decide what kind of realities we are going to construct.

These readings were created as a guide to help you understand the unique power of your mind, your choices, and your impact. It is, essentially, a beginner's "how to" guide for creating realities, although it is by no means the final word on the subject. This book is more like a conversation, as opposed to a "This is how it is" lecture. I use passages and verses as the start, not the end, of a subject or an issue.[8] Like the early followers of the Messiah, I believe that the Bible is a series of narratives that speak to, not rule over, human society.[9]

These readings provide a platform for discussion: every day it is up to you to examine the Scripture in question in an attempt to form a framework for dealing with life. In other words, this verse helps construct a worldview that can create realities of love through reading the Bible and allowing "it to read you."[10] These readings are essentially a way of tapping into the authority of *logos* and manifesting God's love as "flesh" into your life, acting in love, just as Jesus was God's love incarnated. It is about bringing *heaven to earth* through your choices (Deut. 30:19; Matt. 6:11).

Each Scripture will be followed by a "Brainy Tip." Science is not only exciting but also another way of worshiping God. It tells us about his magnificent creation: where Scripture gives us the *why*, science tells us about the *how*.[11] We should not come to Scripture demanding it bow to science or vice versa. Understanding the science behind Scripture is a more holistic and meaningful way of approaching biblical narratives, allowing us to see and understand elements of the text that hitherto went unnoticed. It allows us to approach the text as a dialogue between two very different but often complementary vantage points. This dialogue encourages not only more questions but also an incredible sense of wonder at the magnificence of our Creator. I would go as far as to say that it helps us comprehend how the library of books that make up the Bible can be a "book of the people," one that facilitates community and love between various peoples.[12]

Some concepts are discussed over several days, while some verses are used for more than one day. Repetition is, after all, necessary for the protein synthesis and consolidation of memory! Each new reading will cover a different aspect of the verse, allowing you to read and think deeply about what it has to say and how it can impact your life. In the rabbinic tradition, each verse of Scripture is said to be like a jewel: every time you turn the surface, light is reflected in a different way.[13] Every time you look at a verse from a different angle, you see something unique and beautiful, which is why it is important to respect both the context and the complexity of every word, sentence, and passage in the Bible, as I have attempted to do in these readings.

Likewise, certain concepts, such as the power of thinking and choosing, will feature throughout these readings, since they form the backbone of a renewed lifestyle. As leading biblical scholar N. T. Wright notes, the apostle Paul's worldview "will only function if it is held together by humans with transformed minds, and who use those transformed minds constantly to wrestle with the biggest questions of all, those of God and the world."[14] Our ability to think, feel, and choose has the power of life and death and will determine the way we live our lives today and in the new creation.

Following the Scripture and Brainy Tip is the reading of the day. I hope you won't just read it and move on. Rather, I encourage you to get a journal and write in it each day about what you have read. I recommend the following process to your writing: *ask*, *answer*, and *discuss*. These three actions underscore the intentional and deliberate *process* of learning that produces intelligent memory, which goes beyond merely reading some information you will forget at a later date (for more information on learning and memory formation, see my book *Think, Learn, Succeed*).

First, you *ask*. In your journal, write down several questions about the reading. Writing them down will help you start thinking about the verse(s) within the bigger picture of renewing your mind and reflecting God's glory through your thoughts, words, and actions. For example, you can think of questions like "How do you think renewing the mind applies to your life? Can you think of examples in your own life when you had to literally change your mind and how it impacted what you said and/or did? Have you ever felt that you were not good enough? That you could not cope with the circumstances of life? How did you respond? What effect did this have in your life?" Your *ask* section does not, of course, have to cover every aspect of the passage in question—the Bible is a complex series of books that will take many lifetimes to explore. Rather, your *ask* questions are meant to provide a starting point for dialogue, much like questions we ask during our day-to-day conversations.

Next, you *answer*. Here you apply the passage to your own life by responding, in detail, to your questions in the *ask* section. It is important to remember that there are no right or wrong answers in this section—you are talking to the text, thinking about the questions you wrote down, and answering them honestly and realistically. You answer your own questions, which are shaped by your experiences and the unique way you think, feel, and choose (see my book *The Perfect You* for more information).

Finally, you *discuss*. In your journal, you further examine your own thoughts, words, and actions in light of the Bible passage, expanding your observations and discussing ways you can renew your mind and change your life. In effect, you are analyzing your responses in the *answer* section vis-à-vis the Bible verse of the day. If you are reading this book as part of a group study, you can compare your own thoughts and experiences on the text with those of the other members of the group. This approach encourages a natural dialogue with the text, allowing you to come back again, year after year, and discover new ways of reading the Bible that leave you motivated and transformed.

Much of the material in these readings has its foundation in my books *Switch On Your Brain*, *Think and Eat Yourself Smart*, *The Perfect You*, and my latest book, *Think, Learn, Succeed*. If you would like to know more about the many topics covered in this book, and how to practice renewing your mind in a practical way, I would suggest you visit the Dr. Leaf Store at drleaf.com. I also have many talks available on my YouTube channel, and other books and materials available at both drleaf.com and retailers such as Amazon and Barnes & Noble.

One word on Scripture translations. For the Old Testament, I have used the New Revised Standard Version, as it is a fairly accurate translation, both in terms of language and in terms of cultural context. For the New Testament, I have used the *The Kingdom New Testament* by N. T. Wright, one of the leading New Testament scholars in our world today. Wright's translation pays close attention to the historical context of the New Testament Gospels and letters, allowing the reader to step into the world of the first century CE and truly experience the writings of the early followers of the Messiah. You are welcome to use other translations alongside these two versions. You can even translate the Scriptures yourself if desired. Shifting between translations will force you to analyze the Scriptures from a variety of different viewpoints, worldviews, and social nuances, which certainly increases mind health! David Bentley Hart recently came out with an incredible, raw, and intimate translation of the New Testament that I highly recommend as well.

Most important, however, is to remember the power you have in your mind as you work through these readings. Your choices, where you direct your thinking, and what you decide to meditate on, can change the world—for good or for ill. God has given us this incredible power to choose, a reflection of the mind of the divine, so choose life!

Day 1

What's more, don't let yourselves be squeezed into the shape dictated by the present age. Instead, be transformed by the renewing of your minds, so that you can work out what God's will is—what is good, acceptable, and complete.
—Romans 12:2

> **Brainy Tip:** The brain is neuroplastic: it changes according to its environment. What we allow into our brains, through the choices we make with our minds, can change the structure of our brains for good or for bad.

We don't live in a bubble. We live in multifaceted, dynamic environments; each day it seems like there are a thousand voices telling us what we should believe, say, do, and wear. They tell us what life should be like and what we ought to be doing with our time. It is easy to give in to these voices, listening to them and allowing them to take root inside our heads. It is easy to "be squeezed into shape" by whatever is popular today.

But we do have the power to say no. We do have the power to say "This is not who I am. This is not who I want to be." By observing and monitoring what we think about and the choices we make, we can change the structure of our brains, saying no to "the present age," making the Messiah Lord over every area of our lives. We can say yes to his love, his glory—to the way he created us, to the passions he has placed inside us. We have the power to determine the direction of our lives.

Day 2

What's more, don't let yourselves be squeezed into the shape dictated by the present age. Instead, be transformed by the renewing of your minds, so that you can work out what God's will is—what is good, acceptable, and complete.
—*Romans 12:2*

> **Brainy Tip:** Regardless of what has happened to us, or what is happening to us, we can change our brains through our choices! Change takes time, but it is possible.

Building a life of Christian character is an unremitting task, but thankfully our powerful minds are certainly up for the challenge! Each day we can choose to think differently, although we must remember that Rome wasn't built in a day, as the saying goes. True, lasting change takes time and not a little effort. How many times have you tried to change and failed? One of the great things about Romans 12:2 is the word "renewing"—the action is continuous, daily.

Our brains can change, and as we learn to renew the way we think, we change our brains, building Christian character and learning to act and speak like the Messiah. It is really all about learning how to be truly human again, reflecting the image of our glorious Creator. It is not instant—not just one prayer we say and "voila!" we are perfect Christians. Each day, as we choose to follow the Messiah, we change the structure of our brains, a change that in turn impacts our thoughts, words, and actions.

Day 3

What's more, don't let yourselves be squeezed into the shape dictated by the present age. Instead, be transformed by the renewing of your minds, so that you can work out what God's will is—what is good, acceptable, and complete.
—Romans 12:2

> **Brainy Tip:** Where our minds go, our brains follow.

What we have built into our minds through our experiences and choices shapes our unique worldview, which in turn impacts our thoughts, words, and actions. It is our filter, reflecting and refracting what comes in through our senses and shaping our mental architecture. Once we choose to follow the Messiah, however, we have to compare our worldview to God's worldview. We have a beautiful new filter that not only adds to our experiences but paints them in a new light, one that is "good, acceptable, and complete," allowing us to see and respond to the world in a different way—in a truly human way. The more we choose with our minds to think and act like Jesus, the more we become like Jesus. Where our minds go, our brains follow.

Day 4

After all, the spirit given to us by God isn't a fearful spirit;
it's a spirit of power, love, and prudence [a sound mind].
—2 Timothy 1:7

> **Brainy Tip:** We are wired for love. Science shows how we have a natural optimism bias.

So often in life we are told that we do not measure up, that we aren't good enough. Perhaps we even tell ourselves that we will never succeed. Our days are filled with worries, cares, and concerns. We feel overwhelmed. But science and Scripture say otherwise. We are not designed to go through life with a "fearful spirit," not able to cope with or face our problems. We are wired for love: every cell in our body is created to respond to thoughts and feelings of life, wholeness, passion, and truth.

When we choose to follow the Messiah, to follow his rule of love, we are given his "prudence"—his sound mind, which is powerful! We can face whatever life throws our way, because we stand on firm ground. Our experiences will never be perfect, but when we choose to pursue a life of love, victory will always be possible.

Day 5

We take every thought prisoner and make it obey the Messiah.—2 Corinthians 10:5

Brainy Tip: Thoughts are real and occupy mental real estate.

It is nice to think of victory, but how do we *believe* in victory? How do we believe that things can change? It starts in our minds. It is easy to think that thoughts are not really things and don't really impact our health and the quality of our lives. I mean, what is a thought? Isn't it just a bit of hot air? The most important thing is what we do with that thought, right?

Thoughts are real things—when we think on something, we build it into the structure of our brain. A thought is a physical entity, changing the environment of our brain and body. When we choose to allow a thought to grow inside our brains, feeding it with attention and time, it will affect the cells in our brain and body, impacting our future thoughts, words, and actions. It is therefore incredibly important to monitor what we allow in our heads, taking "every thought prisoner" and making sure the things we think about are good and wholesome, not toxic and harmful. We are what we think, so think wisely!

Day 6

*I call heaven and earth to witness against you today that
I have set before you life and death, blessings and curses.
Choose life, so that you and your descendants may live.*
—Deuteronomy 30:19

> **Brainy Tip:** The choices you make impact your health, mentally and physically, and the world around you—through the generations.

This verse is one of my favorites. It is compelling and challenging. We are designed to do our own brain surgery and rewire our brains by thinking and by choosing to renew our minds. It all begins with choice! Our choices can bring life or death, and through epigenetics the impact of these choices can be felt through the generations. We thus live in a community in both the present and future. What we choose today has a lasting impact. This verse compels us to examine our thoughts and ask whether they are life-bearing or death-bearing. It highlights our responsibility as human beings made in the image of a powerful God.

Yet Deuteronomy 30:19 is also incredibly encouraging. Through our thoughts we can be our own micro-surgeons as we make choices that will change the circuits in our brains. So, no matter what "death" we may have faced in the past, we can still choose life. We can choose to change. There is always hope.

Day 7

For the rest, my dear family, these are the things you should think through: whatever is true, whatever is holy, whatever is upright, whatever is pure, whatever is attractive, whatever has a good reputation; anything virtuous, anything praise-worthy.—Philippians 4:8

Brainy Tip: Whatever you think about the most grows.

Have you ever gotten a song stuck in your head? It plays over and over again, and you can't stop singing it. It drives you crazy, but you keep belting out those lyrics. The beat is never-ending. Well, your thinking is kind of like that. The more you think about something, the stronger it grows in your brain. And the stronger it grows, the more influence it has on your future thoughts, words, and actions, even if you don't really like where it is taking you. The more you think about something, the more you "can't stop singing the song," so to speak.

It is incredibly important to monitor your thoughts, making sure that they are true, holy, upright, pure, attractive, of good reputation, virtuous, and praiseworthy. These are the kinds of things you want inside your head—these are the kinds of things that lead to a healthy mind, body, and spirit because they characterize your worldview and shape your choices. These are the kinds of songs you really want to be singing! If you truly want to reflect the glory of God into the world, you need to be very aware of what you are choosing to think about, moment by moment, day after day.

Day 8

A glad heart makes a cheerful countenance.—Proverbs 15:13

Brainy Tip: Smiling is good for your health!

Did you know that the mere act of smiling can stop a negative toxic mindset? In fact, research shows that smiling a lot can rewire the circuit in the brain that helps you keep a positive attitude toward life! This means God has designed us in such a way that when you smile with your eyes and mouth—a real, deep, meaningful smile (called the Duchenne smile)—the part of your brain involved in decision-making, intellectual pursuit, shifting between thoughts, and thinking things through rationally becomes stronger and more effective. Simply put, smiling makes you happier and more intelligent!

And just watch the effect on those around you, because smiling, like an attitude, is contagious. In fact, it's almost impossible not to respond to a real smile: the mirror neurons God has so graciously wired into your brain are designed to respond with a burst of feel-good chemicals that lift your spirits and intellect. Smiling can improve not only your health but the health of people around you. It is a way of reflecting and sharing God's love, so make an effort to smile more.

Day 9

Let the heavens be glad, and let the earth rejoice; let the sea roar, and all that fills it; let the field exult, and everything in it. Then shall all the trees of the forest sing for joy.
—Psalm 96:11–12

> **Brainy Tip:** Laughter and play are incredibly healthy, no matter how old you are!

Incorporating play and laughter into your life is a wonderful way to increase mental and physical wellbeing. In fact, laughing, which is often referred to as "internal jogging," increases the flow of peptides and quantum energy in your brain and body. Many studies show why laughter deserves to be known as "the best medicine." It releases an instant flood of feel-good chemicals that boost the immune system. Almost instantaneously, it reduces levels of stress hormones.

Having fun through laughter and rejoicing is the cheapest, easiest, and most effective way to increase happiness. It rejuvenates the mind, body, and spirit and gets positive emotions flowing. Make an effort to laugh and play more!

Day 10

A cheerful heart is a good medicine, but a downcast spirit dries up the bones.—Proverbs 17:22

Brainy Tip: Your brain and body respond to your mind.

It is important to remember that thoughts create your mood. When you experience a fear-based emotion, you will feel "under the weather" and your thoughts will be shaped by your negativity. Your thinking will become distorted and you will lose the joy of the "now" moment, making your body vulnerable to other diseases and illnesses. Toxic thinking and stress have even been shown to reduce the size of certain structures in the brain.

If, however, your thinking is positive, your mental and physical health will improve. A cheerful heart really is like good medicine, allowing you to pursue your dreams, because your brain and body respond to love. You are, after all, created in the image of a God who is love.

Day 11

Do not eat the bread of the stingy; do not desire their delicacies; for like a hair in the throat, so are they. "Eat and drink!" they say to you; but they do not mean it.—Proverbs 23:6–7

> **Brainy Tip:** Your thoughts change the structure of your brain, which shapes your words and actions. You are what you think.

It seems like everyone has heard of the verse "as a man thinketh, so is he." One of the most famous lines in the King James Version, Proverbs 23:7 has been used in songs, books, and films. So what is all this about a "hair in the throat"? The NRSV translation is closer to the original text, warning us to be careful when a stingy person shows generosity, because "they do not mean it."

The meaning of "throat" in the original Hebrew is something akin to the "inner person," soul, or mind.[1] Within the context of the preceding and following verses, it appears the author is telling us about the importance of not only good actions like generosity and hospitality but also good motives. We have all had those experiences when someone does something nice for us, but there is just something "off" about the situation. It is not just important to do the right thing but also to *think* the right thing, since what we think eventually comes out one way or another and can poison our relationships and our health. No wonder Jesus placed so much emphasis on what is in our hearts!

Day 12

What use will it be, otherwise, if you win the whole world but forfeit your true life [soul/mind/inner being/consciousness]? What will you give to get your life back?—Matthew 16:26

Brainy Tip: What you think about the most will determine the course of your life.

The world is full of people who will tell you what you must do with your life. You should be this, you should do that, you should have so and so many children, you should have a job that pays this much, you should look like this person, you should speak like that person—the list can go on and on and on. It can squeeze the life out of you, and one day you wake up and realize that you did everything you were told to do and are utterly miserable. You allowed all those words and commands to take shape in your mind, changing the structure of your brain and determining the course of your life. And now you hate where your life has ended up.

The good news is that it is never too late to change. It is never too late to say, "No, this is not who I am." When you change your thinking, embracing the wonderful, unique way God made you, you can find happiness, a deep sense of "true life," as you discover what drives you and what gets you out of bed in the morning—regardless of what is happening in your life.

Your brain can always change, because your thinking can always change. You can choose who, or what, you are going to listen to. You can choose who you are going to be.

Day 13

I praise you, for I am fearfully and wonderfully made. Wonderful are your works; that I know very well.—Psalm 139:14

Brainy Tip: We all have a unique way of thinking, feeling, and choosing.

We all have a unique way we think, feel, and choose. We see and process the world differently. We have something exceptional and beautiful to give to the world. We reflect a wonderful, glorious, unique part of the image of God.

If we are not who we are supposed to be, if we have been squeezed, trampled, and changed by what the empires of the world say, if we have become someone we barely recognize or know, we can change. We can rediscover our perfect selves, who we were created to be. We can recognize that we are more than enough, because we are the "wonderful work" of a loving, magnificent God.

Day 14

For the body, indeed, is not one member, but many.—1 Corinthians 12:14

Brainy Tip: We all process information in different ways.

The way we think, feel, and choose allows us to change the world in a unique and wonderful way. It is a gift and a responsibility. We have something to give to the world: our soul, our passion, our "true life." The world is incomplete if we are incomplete or at odds with ourselves. Our communities need us. Our differences are complementary, and as we embrace who we are as well as allow others to be who they are, we can truly learn to love and care for each other and this beautiful world God has entrusted to us.

Day 15

Let the king's peace be the deciding factor in your hearts; that's what you were called to, within the one body. And be thankful.—Colossians 3:15

> **Brainy Tip:** You are able to stand outside yourself, observe your own thinking, consult with God, and change the negative, toxic thought or grow the healthy, positive thought. When you do this, your brain responds with a positive neurochemical rush and structural changes that will improve your intellect, health, and peace. You will experience soul harmony and share that harmony with others.

One of the greatest things about being human is that we can choose, even when times are difficult. We can choose God's life, "the king's peace," and through our thinking implant that peace deep within our nonconscious minds, allowing it to shape the way we react to the people in our lives.

We are not subject to the whims, opinions, or choices of others. Our differences do not need to divide us. Regardless of what other people believe, do, or say, we can respond in love, because that love is planted deep within our inner person. Reacting in this way not only improves our relationships but also our health—mentally and physically.

Day 16

Let the king's peace be the deciding factor in your hearts; that's what you were called to, within the one body. And be thankful. —Colossians 3:15

> **Brainy Tip:** We all think, feel, and choose in different ways. Our differences are complementary—there is no need to compete with others.

We have to deal with people. With their opinions, their choices, our lack of control over what they do . . . even if we don't feel like it. Indeed, one of the apostle Paul's greatest concerns was the unity of the early church. How do we create "one body"? How do we create communities that truly love each other, even if they are all so different? It is great to say we need to love our neighbor, but what if our neighbor is, well, a fool?

Love! We are wired for love, for companionship, and for community. When we recognize that we all think, feel, and choose in different ways, that we all have something beautiful and unique to contribute, we no longer feel the need to compete with each other or disregard our differences. Being "one body" is possible, and when we are who we truly are and others are who they truly are, we can work together, letting God's peace rule, and we can be "thankful" for such a community!

Day 17

"All right," [Jesus] said, "it's time for a break. Come away, just you, and we'll go somewhere lonely [secluded] and private."—Mark 6:31

Brainy Tip: Quality rest is essential for mental wellbeing.

I am sure you have experienced periods in your life when you are so busy you can barely breathe. You run from one task to another, and by the time you get in bed at night (if you even get to bed at all), you feel like you are going to collapse. I certainly know the feeling!

At times like these, it is important to remember that our brains need a good break every now and then. The quality of our quiet time, a time when we go "somewhere lonely and private" and meditate on good things, will contribute to the quality of our mental health. When we direct our rest by introspection, self-reflection, and prayer; when we catch our toxic thoughts; when we study, memorize, and quote Scripture; and when we develop our minds intellectually, we enhance the default mode network (DMN) that improves brain function and mental, physical, and spiritual health.

Day 18

Be still, and know that I am God! I am exalted among the nations, I am exalted in the earth.—Psalm 46:10

Brainy Tip: If you are constantly in busy mode, your mental and physical health will suffer.

There is something so powerful about "being still." We can strive and strive to get things done—there will be times in our lives when we are called to hustle and work hard—but there are also times in our lives when we have to learn to say no. No, we will not be pressured into doing something. No, we will not let our circumstances burn us out, because God is greater than whatever we are facing in our lives. No, we will not let life get the better of us; we will not let whatever we are going through make us sick, depressed, and tired.

Rest, partnered with gratitude and the realization that God's love is on our side, can help us maintain a sense of peace during turbulent times. It can help us choose life, even when it seems we are surrounded by pain, suffering, and death. It can give us the strength to carry on, to fight the good fight. It can help maintain our mental and physical wellbeing. It is a time of restoration and renewal, giving us the energy to face the next day with a smile on our face.

Day 19

*So put away everything that is sordid, all that overflowing
malice, and humbly receive the word which has been planted
within you and which has the power to rescue your lives.*
—James 1:21

> **Brainy Tip:** What you wire into your brain through thinking is
> stored in your nonconscious mind. The nonconscious mind is
> where 99.9 percent of our mind activity is. It is the root level that
> stores the thoughts with the emotions and perceptions, and it im-
> pacts the conscious mind and what we say and do.

As I mentioned before, you are what you think. What you
choose to focus on, what you choose to think about, will
change the structure of your brain. So if you choose to worry
about something, thinking about it on a daily basis, you build
this concern into your nonconscious mind, which then impacts the way you think, feel, and choose. Essentially, you
have built a worldview of fear, which shapes the way you
react to the world.

Yet when you choose to follow the Messiah, you "put away"
all these negative thoughts. On a daily basis, you choose to
renew your mind, taking your thoughts captive and meditating on what is good and beautiful. And the more you meditate
on these good things, the more you "plant" the worldview of
Jesus deep within you. When you start seeing the world from
the Messiah's angle, you see the truth of your humanity and
the power of love, which has "the power to rescue our lives."

Day 20

Someone living at the merely human level doesn't accept the things of God's spirit. They are foolishness to such people, you see, and they can't understand them because they need to be discerned spiritually. But spiritual people discern everything, while nobody else can discern the truth about them! For "Who has known the mind of the Lord, so as to instruct him?" But we have the mind of the Messiah.—1 Corinthians 2:14–16

Brainy Tip: What we listen to and think about changes the structure of our brains.

We have all faced moments when following the way of Jesus seemed foolish. I mean, loving our enemies? Turning the other cheek? Forgiving the people who hurt us or those we love? We want to make people pay. It makes more sense than letting them get away with it, right? It is about justice, right?

Repaying evil in kind, however, never really works out in the end. It can spiral out of control as each person attacks the other, and can continue on for years and even decades. Justice and violence are not interchangeable terms. We can fight fire with fire, as the saying goes, but we do run the risk of getting burned. In fact, bitterness and uncontrolled anger can hurt us as much as they hurt the person we are trying to get even with.

Loving those who are hard to love may sound ridiculous, but if we want to see a different kind of world, one where love, mercy, compassion, humility, and grace run the show, then perhaps reacting in a more loving way makes sense. Perhaps, instead of sending in the tanks, we can send in the meek, the humble, and the peacemakers, and see a different, surprisingly wonderful result. Now, wouldn't that be something?

Day 21

Someone living at the merely human level doesn't accept the things of God's spirit. They are foolishness to such people, you see, and they can't understand them because they need to be discerned spiritually. But spiritual people discern everything, while nobody else can discern the truth about them! For "Who has known the mind of the Lord, so as to instruct him?" But we have the mind of the Messiah.—1 Corinthians 2:14–16

> **Brainy Tip:** We have the power to create realities using our minds. We can bring life into the world through our thoughts, feelings, and choices. We have the powerful mind of the Messiah.

When we choose to follow Jesus, who is love, with the help of the Holy Spirit, we can start thinking in a different way—in a more loving way. We have "the mind of the Messiah"! We start to see the world from a different angle, we plant these thoughts deep into our nonconscious mind, and we choose to react differently. The more we act according to God's wisdom, and not how the world says we should, the more we think and act like Jesus.

And, suddenly, what was foolish is not so foolish anymore. We begin to understand that we have the power to create realities of love through what we plant into our heads, which then determine what we say and do. The "way of the world" doesn't seem to be so wise anymore—after thousands and thousands of years, we still have so much suffering, greed, and hatred. We understand that something has to change. We see that making the world a better place starts with our thinking, feeling, and choosing. We essentially learn how to be human again; we learn how to bring heaven, not hell, to earth.

Day 22

May your kingdom come, may your will be done as in heaven, so on earth.—Matthew 6:10

Brainy Tip: Our thoughts change our brain, impacting our health and the world around us.

We are God's masterpieces, created in his image. We are designed to reflect his glory into the world. We were created to bring heaven to earth.

This all sounds wonderfully grand, of course, but how do we do this? How do we bring heaven to earth, as the Lord's Prayer says? What does this look like as we go about our daily activities?

When we start to think with the mind of the Messiah, renewing our minds and taking thoughts captive with the help of the Holy Spirit, we change our worldview to one of love—to the worldview of heaven. And as we plant this way of thinking deep into our nonconscious minds by directing our attention and meditating on the Word, we change the structure of our brains in a positive direction. This transformation affects our future thoughts, words, and actions, which impact our environment as we interact with the world around us. In effect, we bring heaven to earth! Being truly human is essentially about colonizing the world with the culture of heaven, which we can do because we are created in the image of God.

Day 23

So God created humankind in his image, in the image of God he created them, male and female he created them.
—Genesis 1:27

> **Brainy Tip:** Our thoughts, words, and actions change the world around us. We were created to reflect the image of a magnificent, loving God into the world.

At almost every church conference I speak at, I hear at least one person say excitedly that we are "made in the image of God." It certainly is a powerful statement. Yet what exactly does it mean for the way we speak and act? What power do our words and actions have? What power do our thoughts have, if they are the foundation of what we do and say?

We are designed to show the world God's love; we are designed to reflect his loving image into the world and reflect the praises of creation back to God. We are his "angled mirrors."[1] When we think, feel, and choose according to our design, we show the world who God truly is. But when we constantly think negative thoughts, which in turn impact our words and actions, we do not reflect the image of a loving God into the world; we reflect a broken image.

It is therefore incredibly important to monitor what we are thinking, feeling, and choosing. We have the power to choose, no matter what we have done or what has been done to us. We can choose to think like God, reflecting his image into our world, thereby living the way we were created to live. Being made in the image of God truly is a magnificent truth and a reminder of both our power and our responsibility!

Day 24

The one who does not love has not known God, because God is love.—1 John 4:8

> **Brainy Tip:** We are wired for love. This statement is known as the optimism bias in science. Loving others is built into our natural design, which brings health, healing, and joy.

Choice is an integral part of love—love cannot exist without the freedom of choice, and God's love for us has given us the power to choose. We have the power to choose life or death, blessings or curses. We are created in the image of God "who is love," but we can still choose what sort of image we want to reflect into the world. Through the thoughts we build into our brain, which shape our future thoughts, words, and actions, we create the type of world we want to see.

We need to look deep into our inner person—the nonconscious mind. What kind of worldview do we have planted there? Does it need to change? Do we fail to love others? Do we truly know the Creator, whose loving image we bear? Do we feel at odds with ourselves, mentally and physically? I know I, for one, do not always act in love (especially when the grocery store lines are long and the person at the register is taking forever!).

Yet when we choose to take our thoughts captive and renew our minds, activating the wired-for-love design of our brain and body, we will learn to act, and react, in love. As a result, we will embrace our true identity as image-bearers of a God who is love. We will feel at peace within ourselves, which will give us a deep, rich sense of physical and mental wellbeing; we are acting like we should, since we are wired to love.

Day 25

Indeed, he is actually not far from each one of us, for in him we live and move and exist; as also some of your own poets have put it, "For we are his offspring."—Acts 17:27–28

Brainy Tip: Consciousness upholds the universe: God's mind, or *logos*, the supreme consciousness, is the source of all existence. Since God is love, the whole world is wired for love and held together in love.

As I mentioned in the introduction to these readings, elementary particles like atoms and electrons are not necessarily actual "things." These particles form a world of possibilities, which are made into actualities through the choices of the observer. Essentially, the whole of reality is a construct of the mind of the observer. And since God is always observing and always present, he is the ultimate reality. Through him all things have their existence.

If God is love, as we saw yesterday, then love underpins the universe. Love is the reason we "live and move and exist." When we act according to this loving design, we experience God in a personal and wonderful way, and we get to know the Creator whose image we bear and reflect. We act according to our natural, wired-for-love design—the key component for a healthy lifestyle!

Day 26

There is no faithfulness or loyalty, and no knowledge of God in the land. Swearing, lying, and murder, and stealing and adultery break out; bloodshed follows bloodshed. Therefore the land mourns, and all who live in it languish; together with the wild animals and the birds of the air, even the fish of the sea are perishing. —Hosea 4:1–3

Brainy Tip: We live in an entangled world. What we think, say, and do affect not only us but everyone and everything around us.

Almost every day I read something about climate change. It reminds me how much of an impact we have on the world. What we do has ripple effects. Our thoughts, words, and actions affect the people we know and love, and everything around us. Quantum physicists describe this interdependence as "entanglement." Entanglement is found throughout the Bible. We are stewards of the world and have a responsibility to reflect God's loving image into creation.

If, however, we do not act as responsible stewards, "the land mourns." Animals, birds, fish, and every living thing suffers because of human greed, violence, and corruption. Think of wars. What happens to the land? Think of human greed. How does it affect natural disasters? It is therefore incredibly important that we monitor what we think, which forms our mindset: the way we see and interact with the world. We were created to bring heaven, not hell, to earth. We have to think about how we can engage with the world in a loving, productive way.

Day 27

Yes: creation itself is on tiptoe with expectation, eagerly awaiting the moment when God's children will be revealed. Creation, you see, was subjected to pointless futility, not of its own volition, but because of the one who placed it in this subjection, in the hope that creation itself would be freed from its slavery to decay, to enjoy the freedom that comes when God's children are glorified.—Romans 8:19–21

Brainy Tip: The mind is powerful: thoughts are the roots of words and actions, which can change the world—for good or ill.

We live in an entangled world, so what we think, feel, and choose affects the whole of creation. We bear the image of God, so we are responsible for how we steward that image—we are responsible for how we use the power of choice he has given us.

When we sin, which essentially means "missing the mark/target" of being human, we do not use his image wisely, and our toxic choices bring "slavery and decay" to the whole world.[1] Life is "subjected to a pointless futility" because we have given up the glory of our Creator.

When we choose to follow the Messiah, however, thinking with his mind and embracing a lifestyle of love, we reflect God's glory back into the world. Indeed, creation is "eagerly awaiting the moment" when we finally get our act together and start acting as human beings ought to act, as wise, glory-bearing stewards. It is therefore imperative that we change the way we think, in order that we may be truly, wonderfully human.

Day 28

For in him all the Fullness was glad to dwell and through him to reconcile all to himself, making peace through the blood of his cross, through him—yes, things on the earth, and also the things in the heavens.—Colossians 1:19–20

> **Brainy Tip:** Our thoughts, words, and actions have the power to create realities—this is literal "genesis" power.

I think that one of the gloomiest notions some Christians have is the desire to get to heaven soon, since the earth is going to be destroyed anyway. They see the apocalypse as something terrible: lakes of fires, unending pain, disasters, and all sorts of horrors. The word *apocalypse*, however, just means "unveiling."[1] Just as the veil was torn when Jesus died, the veil between heaven, God's realm, and earth will be pulled back, and we will see creation how it was always intended to be seen.

That doesn't mean we can't see heaven on earth right now, in the present. As Paul notes in Colossians 1, all things "on the earth" and "in the heavens" have been reconciled to God through the Messiah. The kingdom of God is "now, not yet."[2] When Jesus rose again, he was victorious over death, over fear, over every terrible thing in our world. We are living in the in-between phase of victory and completion, and everything we think, say, or do will either be for the kingdom or not. Our thoughts, words, and actions today have eternal significance. We serve God in order that his kingdom will be unveiled in the present—in the *now*. We really need to think, choose, and feel very wisely, because we create realities in the present with our thoughts!

Day 29

Yours, O LORD, are the greatness, the power, the glory, the victory, and the majesty; for all that is in the heavens and on the earth is yours; yours is the kingdom, O LORD, and you are exalted as head above all.—1 Chronicles 29:11

Brainy Tip: The whole world is wired for love.

The world was created by a God who is love. We are made in the image of a God who is love, entrusted with caring for his creation. What we think, and hence what we say and do, is designed to reflect God's love into the world, since the world is his. The foundation of the whole world is love!

Sir Roger Penrose, an Oxford mathematician, has created complex calculations indicating that love is embedded in space-time in "ingredient" form.[1] As we humans choose, we can access these love ingredients to think and function in love through what we say and do. However, through our choices we can also distort these love-based probabilities and produce toxicity in our environment.

It is our duty to choose wisely. We are tasked with bringing heaven to earth. What we think, say, and do has global repercussions. We have to think beyond "me, myself, and I" and ask ourselves, *What does love look like in community and the global perspective?*

Day 30

If someone already has something, you see, they will be given more, and they'll have plenty. But if someone has nothing, even what they have will be taken away from them.
—Matthew 25:29

> **Brainy Tip:** The ability to think and create with our thoughts is not only a gift but also a responsibility—thoughts are the roots of our words and actions, which produce fruit in our life.

We should take our roles as stewards of creation seriously. As in the parable of the talents, God has given us the world to take care of, and when he returns he will ask us how we have stewarded not only our own lives but also his beautiful world.

If Jesus stood before you today, what would you say about your stewardship of your spirit, mind, brain, body, and the world we live in? Do you take what you need and use what you have for your own pleasure or for God's glory? The way you live your life is a reflection of the way you love your God.

Day 31

The LORD is good to all, and his compassion is over all that he has made.—Psalm 145:9

> **Brainy Tip:** As sentient beings, we need to choose, on a daily basis, to care for and have compassion for not only our minds and bodies but also the whole world.

God cares for *everything* he has made. His love for creation is reflected throughout the Bible. As human beings made in the image of this loving, merciful, and gracious God, we ought to have compassion for the whole of creation. As human beings, we need to think about how our thoughts, words, and actions impact the world around us and how we can reflect the glorious love of God into the world.

It is easy to sit back and complain about how bad the world is, but as the high priests of creation we cannot afford to spend our lives moaning about how things should be. We are designed to reflect the perfect love of God into the world with our thinking. We have the power to give life. We will be held accountable for how we use this power.

Day 32

The earth is the LORD's and all that is in it, the world, and those who live in it; for he has founded it on the seas, and established it on the rivers.—Psalm 24:1–2

Brainy Tip: We live in an entangled world that has love as its basic reality.

It certainly is nice to think that we are sons and daughters of the Most High God. At every conference I go to, at least one person sings about "the children of God" and "sons and daughters of the King." But what does it actually mean to be God's children? How does it change the way we live our lives?

Everything was created by God—it all belongs to him. As his children, his high priests, we are called to reflect the Father's glory into the world by taking care of what is his. We are called to sum up the praises of creation in him.[1] Yet if our thinking is toxic, we cannot reflect God's love into the world. If we do not renew our minds, we cannot change our lives or the lives of anyone around us. We cannot truly be children of God unless we love what God loves.

Day 33

In his hand is the life of every living thing and the breath of every human being.—Job 12:10

> **Brainy Tip:** Compassion and love heal the brain and body. This compassion and love are things we activate through our choices.

Because everything was created in and through God, creation is dependent on God's sustaining love. This means that the contents of consciousness, or mind, are sustained by God. God is the source of all consciousness; he is truth; he is the supreme consciousness.

As people who bear the image of this consciousness, we have a particular and lasting effect on the world, on each other, and on ourselves. I cannot say this enough: we were created to reflect the glory of God into the world and reflect the praises of creation back to God, but we cannot do this to the best of our abilities if our lives are a mess.

So how do we change? How do we heal? True love breeds compassion, and these two things have the power to heal not only the world but our own brains and bodies. When we embrace the loving and compassionate lifestyle of Jesus, we transform our minds and bodies, healing ourselves and lengthening our own lifespan! This is truly God's grace in action.

Day 34

As for me, I am establishing my covenant with you and your descendants after you, and with every living creature that is with you, the birds, the domestic animals, and every animal of the earth with you, as many as came out of the ark.
—Genesis 9:9–10

Brainy Tip: What we believe shapes how we think, speak, and act.

After the flood in Genesis, God made a covenant with the *whole* world. He promised that he wouldn't destroy creation again—he cares for every living thing. As human beings made in the image of God and as recipients of his covenant, which was fulfilled with the coming of Jesus, we too have a responsibility to care for every living thing.

It is also important to remember why God sent the flood in the first place: sin, or "missing the mark" of being human. At the time, human beings forgot whose image they were made in, choosing to love their idols, destroy the world, and bring hell to earth by pursuing their desires regardless of the cost. If we truly want to be a part of God's covenant, we have to choose, on a daily basis, to bring heaven to earth with our thoughts, words, and actions. We have to choose to renew our minds, operate in love, take negative thoughts captive, and let the Holy Spirit guide our minds, all of which shape how we interact with the world.

Day 35

Six days you shall do your work, but on the seventh day you shall rest, so that your ox and your donkey may have relief.—Exodus 23:12

Brainy Tip: Like every living thing, we need to rest.

In our modern world, ceasing our day-to-day activity is almost a revolutionary idea. Our culture tells us *more, more, more*. We need more money, more cars, more houses, more holidays, more clothes, more time. It is all about consumption, even the consumption of human beings (think of human trafficking).

The kingdom of heaven, however, is about stewardship. Wise stewards do not just take from the world or even from themselves. They give. They respond in love, they understand that quantity is not everything, and they recognize the need for rest, not only for themselves but also for every living thing, including the "ox and donkey."

As image-bearers of God, we have to be aware of the way we treat ourselves *and* the created world. We need to think about *how we think* about creation. Contrary to what the empires of the world may say, it is not all about "me, myself, and I" or "more, more, more." The idea of relief is important because it teaches us not only to rest in the modern sense but also to *respect* every living thing, including our own brains and bodies, which are designed to rest.

Day 36

But the Lord's day will come like a thief. On that day the heavens will pass away with a great rushing sound, the elements will be dissolved in fire, and the earth and all the works on it will be disclosed.—2 Peter 3:10

Brainy Tip: Our minds are the most powerful things in the universe after God.

Many people think that when Jesus comes back, the earth will be consumed by fire and everything will be new again. Unfortunately, that notion is based off a mistranslation from the King James Version of 2 Peter 3:10. The earth will not be burned up but rather "disclosed" or "laid bare" or "found." The underlying Greek word comes from the word for *foundry*, a place where metals were rid of impurities through fire.[1] Essentially, every bad thing that is not of love will be burned up and disappear, but all that is good and beautiful and true will remain. The earth that we know and that many of us love is here to stay, only it will be more perfect than we could ever imagine.

We therefore have to be careful how we treat not only other people but the whole of creation. We need to renew our minds on a daily basis, because our choices have the power of life and death. We bring heaven, or hell, to earth.

And it is certainly encouraging to remember that the love-based thoughts we build into our minds and the good fruit they produce in our lives have eternal significance—they will not be burned up in the new creation!

46

Day 37

He must be received in heaven, you see, until the time which God spoke about through the mouth of his holy prophets from ancient days, the time when God will restore all things.—Acts 3:21

Brainy Tip: It is possible to heal the mind, the brain, and the body. We can retell our story and change our future. We can change the impact that the past has on us. This is called retroactive causation in quantum physics.

Sometimes, looking at the world around us, or even looking at our own lives, it seems that things will never change. The world will always be a mess, and our lives will always be a mess. We will always be sick, tired, and sad.

But you can choose to believe that everything will always stay the same, or you can choose to believe that things can change. That change is possible. You can choose to believe in God's promise that he will restore "all things" under heaven and earth. God can, and will, restore your own life and the world around you. True healing is not only possible with God but promised by God! Remember, God is not bound by time—the ingredients of your future already exist.

Yet you have to choose to believe this healing is possible. You decide what kind of world you want to live for; you decide what kind of reality you are going to create. You can retell your story—you are not bound by your past.

Day 38

But the earth will be filled with the knowledge of the glory of the LORD, as the waters cover the sea.—Habakkuk 2:14

Brainy Tip: You shape your world with your thoughts.

Have you ever felt yourself wondering what everything will be like in the end? What the world will look like when King Jesus returns? Whenever you think, act, and speak in love, and whenever you receive love, you experience a piece of God's glory, a moment of heaven on earth.

But how? Why? We bear the image of God. We are designed to reflect his glory into the world through what we think, say, and do. We can only reflect God's glory, however, if our minds are renewed and transformed in the "knowledge" of his love. When we renew our minds we are able to bring heaven to earth, healing communities and covering the world with his glory, "as the waters cover the sea"! We can live in the present and imagine the future, a future where everything will be beautiful, pure, and good under God. This is our hope, which is everlasting and eternal: a world saturated with the perfect love of the Creator.

Day 39

For the LORD will comfort Zion; he will comfort all her waste places, and will make her wilderness like Eden, her desert like the garden of the LORD; joy and gladness will be found in her, thanksgiving and the voice of song.—Isaiah 51:3

> **Brainy Tip:** Everything we think, say, or do changes our world. Thoughts are real things, made of proteins. Thoughts are not just "hot air."

God promises to heal and comfort not only us but also the entire world. He hears the cries of all living things, and he promises to heal their pain, bringing "joy and gladness" into all of creation—through us. Through us. This is the responsibility of having powerful minds that effect change. We are powerful change agents who can activate love, which brings healing into the world.

As children of God, as agents of this perfect love, we are tasked with bringing his comfort to everyone and everything. We are tasked with using our thoughts, and thus our words and actions, as tools of change, bringing heaven to earth every hour of every day.

Day 40

The LORD God took the man and put him in the garden of Eden to till it and keep it.—Genesis 2:15

Brainy Tip: The way we treat the world around us reflects the worldview we have built into our heads.

If what we say and do is a reflection of what we have built into our minds, how we "keep" creation reflects how we view both our role as human beings and how we view our Creator. God created us to be stewards of the world: to tend to and care for the garden, and to use our free will to benefit the whole world by making it a beautiful place, filled with life and love.

When we misuse the gift of stewardship, however, or when we consume creation rather than care for it, we bring death and destruction into the world. Our minds are powerful; we can bring heaven or hell to earth. We have to take the responsibility that comes with a powerful mind seriously and ask ourselves, on a daily basis: *Am I reflecting God's glory into the world?* Will our thoughts, words, and actions last into the new creation, or will they be burned up?

Day 41

Don't be misled; God won't have people turning their noses up at him. What you sow is what you'll reap. —Galatians 6:7

> **Brainy Tip:** You become what you think about the most. How you choose to use your powerful mind has consequences. This truth is called causal efficacy in science.

Whatever you think about the most grows, shaping the way you see and interact with your environment. This is your "love" in action. When you focus on something constantly and intentionally, you love and "worship" it, giving it power over your mind and your life. As quantum physicist Henry Stapp notes,

> The free choices made by the human players can be seen as miniature versions of the choices that appear to be needed at the creation of the universe. . . . This situation is concordant with the idea of a powerful God that creates the universe and its laws to get things started, but then bequeaths part of this power to beings created in his own image, at least with regard to their power to make physically efficacious decisions on the basis of reasons and evaluations.[1]

The seeds you plant in your head will determine what kind of decisions you make and what you harvest in your life, regardless of your circumstances. You have the power to choose what kind of reality you want to create with your thoughts: one based on the beautiful love of heaven or the toxic lies of the enemy.

Day 42

So, then, whether you eat or drink or whatever you do, do everything to God's glory.—1 Corinthians 10:31

Brainy Tip: We are wired to think and speak and act in a way that optimizes love.

Our brains, bodies, and the world around us were created by a God who is love—a God whose glory is love. Remember, we are designed to act, and react, in true love; we are designed, as image-bearers of God, to reflect his glory into the world.

This love ought to characterize every area of our life: from what we decide to eat to who we choose to be friends with or where we choose to work. We should, on a daily basis, ask the Holy Spirit to guide our thoughts, words, and actions, saturating our communities with the culture of heaven. This kind of love truly makes the world go around.

Day 43

If my people who are called by my name humble themselves, pray, seek my face, and turn from their wicked ways, then I will hear from heaven, and will forgive their sin and heal their land.—2 Chronicles 7:14

Brainy Tip: Our brains and bodies thrive in an environment of love.

The world is, of course, full of problems. There is so much pain, suffering, sickness, and poverty. It sometimes feels as if nothing will change, as if the issues we face have no solution.

Yet there is *hope*. We have a powerful ability to choose what we think about, and thus what we say and what we do. We can be incredible change agents; we can choose to follow the Messiah, renewing our minds and participating in his restoration of *all* things under heaven and on earth. Science, as I mentioned at the beginning of this book, shows us the *how* of operating in true or distorted love and the impact of operating in true or distorted love. We can be a part of God's rescue mission to heal the land and its people.

Indeed, as we serve our communities in love, we heal our own minds. Love is the most powerful healing force. True love is not only a miracle but also creates miracles—true love has a "pay it forward" snowball effect. It is the key to a life of happiness, health, and peace for everyone and everything.

Day 44

Look! I am coming soon. I will bring my reward with me, and I will pay everyone back according to what they have done.—Revelation 22:12

> **Brainy Tip:** You cannot escape your thoughts because you have built them into your brain. Whatever you think about the most grows and gains sufficient quantum energy to impact your next choice and your behavior.

Thoughts are not just thoughts. They are the seeds you plant in your life; they are the reality you choose to embrace; they are the root of your every action and word. You, with your brilliant, creative mind, determine what you think, what you say, what you feel, and what you do. You do not live in a matrix. You are free to think and to be.

When you choose to plant healthy seeds in your mind, you reap a healthy life—and vice versa. Of course, choosing to live a life of love does not mean your life will be perfect and without any mountains to climb, since in many cases you do not control what happens to you. Nevertheless, you can control *how* you react to life by planting seeds of love deep into your mind.

Remember, your reactions will shape your reality. As human beings, we cannot escape the power, and the responsibility, of choice.

Day 45

But you shall keep my statutes and my ordinances and commit none of these abominations, either the citizen or the alien who resides among you (for the inhabitants of the land, who were before you, committed all of these abominations, and the land became defiled); otherwise the land will vomit you out for defiling it, as it vomited out the nation that was before you.—Leviticus 18:26–28

Brainy Tip: We treat our neighbors according to what we believe, which impacts not only other people but also our own brains and bodies.

If we constantly think about our own desires and needs, we make our own image our god. We sacrifice the needs and desires of other people, of every living thing, to this god, "defiling" the image of love in which we were created, bringing destruction and pain into the world and into our brains and bodies.

If, however, we renew our minds and change our thinking, seeing the world as God's beautiful creation and treating others as valued and dignified beings, we heal the world and ourselves. Research has indicated that by helping others, we speed up our own healing by more than 60 percent! We rediscover our true nature as human beings created in the image of a loving, gracious, wonderful God, and we step into our perfect, whole selves.

Day 46

You shall not defile the land in which you live, in which I also dwell; for I the LORD dwell among the Israelites.
—Numbers 35:34

Brainy Tip: How we treat the world we live in is shaped by our thoughts, which form our attitude and worldview.

God is always watching: he sees everything and he upholds all existence as *logos*. He was there before time began; through him and by his love the whole world came into being. He is ever-present; he knows our innermost thoughts, our every word; he dwells among us.

We should constantly be renewing our minds, taking our thoughts captive and choosing love, since we are wired for love. We are wired to tap into the divine reality of God that dwells among us. We are designed to latch on to God's love.

If we don't operate in a loving, respectful way toward all of creation, we defile not only ourselves but the earth as well. If we ignore our wired-for-love design, we forget who we truly are, choosing foolishly and bringing pain and chaos into the world. Think of the effects of manmade climate change, for example, and its impact on every living thing on a global scale.

Yet if we choose to follow the Messiah, we build a relationship with God—becoming our true selves and changing the world for the better. We bring the culture and beauty of heaven to earth, creating little Edens wherever we live.

Day 47

You see, even when we arrived in Macedonia, we couldn't relax or rest. We were troubled in every way; there were battles outside and fears inside.—2 Corinthians 7:5

> **Brainy Tip:** Stress can be good for us, if we choose to react correctly to the circumstances of life.

If I am wired for love, I can't feel any negative emotions, right? I can't be stressed, worried, or fearful, yes? The whole world is counting on me to be happy and loving all the time? Not at all! You can see that even the apostle Paul felt "troubled in every way" at times. Life certainly can be challenging and stressful, with many "battles outside and fears inside"!

The key to making stress work for you is what I call "freaking out in the love zone." Stress can be good for us, depending on how we react to the problems we face. Rather than burying our emotions, which is harmful for our health, we need to learn to deal with them—we need to see our problems with God's eyes. If we have the mind of the Messiah, we don't need to be overwhelmed by what we face. We see the challenge, but we know that God is bigger than that challenge, or any challenge we may face. We know that our minds are powerful enough to handle what comes our way.

Day 48

I don't understand what I do. I don't do what I want, you see, but I do what I hate.—Romans 7:15

Brainy Tip: It takes time and effort to change the way we think, feel, and choose.

I think we all, at some point in our lives, feel like the person St. Paul talks about in Romans 7. We are desperate to do the right thing, but we fail—again and again. How do we change? How do we find the strength to change? Will things ever get better?

It is always important to remember that true change takes time and quite a bit of effort. It takes twenty-one days to build a long-term memory and redesign neural pathways, and another forty-two days to give these new thought networks sufficient energy to become a habit that will impact your behavior. Most people give up after only four or five days, because they don't know or understand the science behind effective, lasting change. But this doesn't have to be you! Don't give up, and "run the race" for at least sixty-three days! Keep reminding yourself that observable change takes up to sixty-three or even eighty-four days, and with each day that passes the structure of your brain is being transformed for the better!

Day 49

What will happen, though, is that you will receive power when the holy spirit comes upon you. Then you will be my witnesses in Jerusalem, in all Judaea and Samaria, and to the very ends of the earth.—Acts 1:8

Brainy Tip: With the help and guidance of the Holy Spirit, we can change the structure of our brains.

The great thing about following the Messiah is that we don't have to do it alone. He has given us the Holy Spirit to help us renew our minds and change our lives, so that we can truly be his witnesses "to the very ends of the earth," bringing heaven to earth through our thoughts, words, and actions. The Holy Spirit is the very breath of heaven on earth—I like to call this "loveness," which we access through our choices.

No matter what you have gone through or are going through, the Holy Spirit can help you if you choose to allow him to help you. He can give you the strength to renew your mind, take your thoughts captive, and change the structure of your brain, healing your past, giving you hope for the future and a deep sense of wellbeing.

Day 50

People whose lives are determined by human flesh focus their minds on matters to do with the flesh, but people whose lives are determined by the spirit focus their minds on matters to do with the spirit.—Romans 8:5

Brainy Tip: Whatever you focus on the most grows.

The Holy Spirit doesn't force us to listen to him. As I keep reiterating: we have to choose, on a daily basis, to let him help us and guide us. We have to choose to "focus our minds" on what he is saying, the "matters to do with the spirit," seeing the world through God's loving eyes. Love demands great freedom; choice gives us that freedom, yet choice has inescapable consequences.

Remember, whatever we think about the most grows and determines the course of our thoughts, words, and actions—the course of our lives. When we choose with our minds to listen to and follow the Holy Spirit, our lives change for the better as we learn to become more and more like the Messiah, reflecting God's glory into the world. With the freedom of love comes great responsibility to choose well, which is why we need to listen to the Spirit of God.

Day 51

My prayer is this: that he will lay out all the riches of his glory to give you strength and power, through his spirit, in your inner being; that the king may make his home in your hearts, through faith; that love may be your root, your firm foundation; and that you may be strong enough (with all God's holy ones) to grasp the breadth and length and height and depth, and to know the king's love—though actually it's so deep that nobody can really know it! So may God fill you with all his fullness.—Ephesians 3:16–19

Brainy Tip: We are designed to be in constant communication with the Spirit of God, who is love. We are designed to be consumed by love, which activates our brain, allowing us to function at our best.

We all have "discomfort zones," times when we just know deep down inside that something isn't right. This could be a flicker of awareness, your heart pounding and adrenaline pumping, or a conflict in your mind as you choose. Maybe it is about something someone said or did, or even about something you did or are thinking of doing. We almost feel as if we just ate something bad—queasy, ill at ease.

These feelings are promptings from the Holy Spirit and a reminder for you to speak to him and ask for his wisdom on a daily basis—both when things are going well and when things are going badly. He can help you take your thoughts captive, renew your mind, and make God your King, Lord over every area of your life.

Day 52

My prayer is this: that he will lay out all the riches of his glory to give you strength and power, through his spirit, in your inner being; that the king may make his home in your hearts, through faith; that love may be your root, your firm foundation; and that you may be strong enough (with all God's holy ones) to grasp the breadth and length and height and depth, and to know the king's love—though actually it's so deep that nobody can really know it! So may God fill you with all his fullness.—Ephesians 3:16–19

Brainy Tip: We reflect what we think about the most. When we are in constant dialogue with the Holy Spirit, we begin to reflect God's loving image into the world.

It is easy to say you want to love others and treat them right, but in reality it is always more complicated than that. Sometimes people are not so lovable!

Thankfully, with the help of the Holy Spirit, we can change the way we think and thus the way we treat others. As we listen to the Spirit, allowing him to plant God's love deep within us, allowing him to fill us with the fullness of God's love, we can begin to truly love others, regardless of how they treat us. We step into our natural, wired-for-love design!

Take some time to observe yourself and your thinking throughout the day. Is your attitude and what you are saying and doing reflecting God's glory into the world?

Day 53

For once people have been enlightened . . . they've tasted the heavenly gift and have had a share in the holy spirit, and have tasted the good word of God and the powers of the coming age.—Hebrews 6:4–5

Brainy Tip: Constantly renewing the mind is the key for peak happiness, thinking, and health.

With the help of the Holy Spirit, we can renew our minds on a daily basis and truly experience heaven on earth in the present. As we learn to think, feel, and choose like Jesus, we can begin to experience the "powers of the coming age" of the new creation. Our thinking becomes "enlightened" as we see creation the way that the Creator sees it.

We start achieving peak happiness, thinking, and health as we live the way we were intended to live: as glorious images of God on earth. This is a deliberate, intentional, and daily process of change, a race that we have to keep running.

Day 54

But the fruit of the spirit is love, joy, peace, great-heartedness, kindness, generosity, faithfulness, gentleness, self-control.
—Galatians 5:22–23

> **Brainy Tip:** When we act according to the fruit of the Spirit, that is, in our wired-for-love mode, we bring healing and joy not only to our own minds and bodies but to everyone around us. We literally affect the brain chemistry and genetic expression of others!

So what exactly does a renewed mind look like? What does a wired-for-love lifestyle look like on a day-to-day basis?

Our thinking, feeling, and choosing in response to life is a quantum signal that physically moves through the substrate of the brain, using it to store and express what we think via what we say and do. When we allow the Holy Spirit to help us choose the right kind of quantum signals, we store healthy, wired-for-love thoughts in our brains, which impact what we say and do and also the people around us.

When we take our thoughts captive and renew our minds, we essentially plant the fruit of the Spirit deep into our non-conscious mind, which enables us to act with "love, joy, peace, great-heartedness, kindness, generosity, faithfulness, gentleness, and self-control" as we respond to the people and the circumstances of life, whatever they may be.

Day 55

Here's how to do it. Hold on to the same love; bring your innermost lives into harmony; fix your minds on the same object. Never act out of selfish ambition or vanity; instead, regard everybody else as your superior. Look after each other's best interests, not your own.—Philippians 2:2–4

Brainy Tip: We become what we focus on the most. For example, if you stay angry at someone, you will become angry.

When we focus on the love of God, rather than our anger, bitterness, or frustration, we allow him to renew our minds through the Holy Spirit, and we can be living examples of his love on earth. We will learn not to act according to our own selfish interests. Rather, we will take care of each other, truly loving our neighbor by loving God, who is love.

The key is focus: directed attention, taking *all* thoughts captive, and renewing the mind. We become what we focus on the most. When we allow the Holy Spirit to help us change the way we think, feel, and choose, "bringing our innermost lives into harmony" with our wired-for-love design, we truly begin to love our neighbor—we focus on his love, not our fears. We start bringing heaven to earth through our thoughts, words, and actions.

Day 56

You must be perfect, just as your heavenly father is perfect.
—*Matthew 5:48*

Brainy Tip: We are as intelligent and successful as we want to be.

We are created in the image of a God who is perfect. We are created to strive for perfection; our brains actually get better and better the more we use them. We design our brains as we activate the blueprint of our Perfect You nature—who God designed us to be.

We have to realize that intelligence, success, and joy do not just "happen." They are not static, tangible things we receive when we cross some perceived finish line, whether this finish line is a new house, a better paycheck, or a five-star holiday in Bali. True happiness and true success come from striving for perfection in the "now" moments of life and enjoying the process of discovering who we are and why we are here. It's a journey, not just a destination.

Day 57

"The first [commandment]," replied Jesus, "is this: 'Listen, Israel: the Lord your God, the Lord is one; and you shall love the Lord your God with all your heart, and with all your soul, and with all your understanding, and with all your strength.' And this is the second one: 'You shall love your neighbor as yourself.' No other commandment is greater than these."
—Mark 12:29–31

> **Brainy Tip:** We are wired for love. When we love others, our brain changes in a positive direction, which is the natural default mode of the brain.

Loving others is essential, not optional. It is the key factor in our mental and physical wellbeing. When we choose to love God (who is the source of all love) and in turn love others because we love God, we change the structure of our brain in a positive direction, which is in line with our wired-for-love design.

Loving ourselves and loving others allows us to live into the image of God that is within all of us. When we choose to follow the Messiah and embrace his commandments, we are able to live a life of happiness and are able to be at peace within ourselves and at peace with others. Jealousy, envy, unforgiveness, bitterness, hatred, and uncontrolled anger create brain damage; love stimulates brain health. When we choose to make love king over our minds and over our lives, we are able to live up to our full potential and allow others to embrace their full potential as well, reflecting the Creator's glory into creation through what we think, say, and feel.

Day 58

*They knew God, but didn't honor him as God or thank him.
Instead, they learned to think in useless ways, and their unwise heart grew dark. They declared themselves to be wise,
but in fact they became foolish. They swapped the glory of
the immortal God for the likeness of the image of mortal
humans—and of birds, animals, and reptiles. . . . Moreover,
just as they did not see fit to hold on to knowledge of God,
God gave them up to an unfit mind, so that they would behave
inappropriately.—Romans 1:21–23, 28*

Brainy Tip: Where your mind goes, your brain follows: you become
what you think about the most.

What happens when you choose to focus on other things,
ignoring the Holy Spirit? What happens when you love other
things more than following the way of the Messiah?

As you think about something, you build it into the structure of your brain. The more you think about it, the stronger
this structure becomes as you bury it deep inside your nonconscious mind. Now this thought is no longer just a thought: it
is a mindset, a way of seeing the world, that influences your
future thoughts, words, and actions.

If this thought is negative, such as a fear, worry, or addiction, meditating on it gives it power over your life. It essentially
becomes an idol: you no longer reflect "the glory of the immortal God." Your life is now characterized by the thing you
think about the most (what you worship). This is a "disordered
love."[1] God no longer has first place in your life. You lose the enlightened wisdom that comes from listening to the Holy Spirit,
thinking in "useless" ways and making "foolish" decisions.

Day 59

They knew God, but didn't honor him as God or thank him. Instead, they learned to think in useless ways, and their unwise heart grew dark. They declared themselves to be wise, but in fact they became foolish. They swapped the glory of the immortal God for the likeness of the image of mortal humans—and of birds, animals, and reptiles. . . . Moreover, just as they did not see fit to hold on to knowledge of God, God gave them up to an unfit mind, so that they would behave inappropriately.—Romans 1:21–23, 28

Brainy Tip: Your thoughts will shape your behavior.

Many people think of God's judgment as a direct, terrible act. They imagine God like the Greek god Zeus, throwing lightning bolts from the sky at those who disobey him, unless Jesus steps in and saves the day.

As I mentioned in day 27, sin means "missing the mark" of being human. We choose to deny the image of our Creator, forgetting the "knowledge of God," and allowing our minds to pursue other loves, which impacts the way we think and thus what we say and do: we "behave inappropriately." We essentially become dehumanized.

Ultimately, God gives us what we want: he allows us to choose what or who to follow by allowing us to choose what we think about. Sin is really a story of "be careful what you wish for." If you choose to think on something, pursuing it and making it lord over your life, God "gives you up to an unfit mind," which impacts your mental and physical well-being and how you interact with the world.

Day 60

Don't you know that a little yeast works its way through the whole lump of dough?—1 Corinthians 5:6

Brainy Tip: Thoughts are real things; they have mental real estate, which means that as we think we create structural change in the brain!

What you think about is built into your brain. Thoughts have *real* mental real estate. They impact your future thoughts and perceptions. They can influence what you think, say, and do. Thoughts, as the roots of actions or words, are very real and ought to be taken very seriously.

If you allow a thought to take root in your head, if you give it energy by thinking about it on a daily basis, it can spread, just like "a little yeast" in a lump of dough. Slowly but surely, this thought can impact your behavior and negatively influence your community. It can spread like a virus and, before you know it, your whole life can take a turn for the worse. Taking your thoughts captive should not, therefore, be optional. It is something that you should practice every moment of every day. Remember, no thought is harmless and no attitude can be hidden.

Day 61

Nobody can serve two masters. Otherwise, they will either hate the first and love the second, or be devoted to the first and despise the second. You can't serve both God and wealth.
—Matthew 6:24

> **Brainy Tip:** Your brain is designed to focus attention on one task at a time.

Our brain can only truly focus on one thing at a time: multi-tasking is a myth. We may feel that we can switch back and forth between one task and another, or focus on many different things at once, but this way of thinking can impede our ability to understand, affecting our mental health.

So, if we are constantly focusing on our own problems or desires, we do not have time to focus on following the Messiah. We focus on what is most important to us and, by focusing on it, are in effect serving this thought, giving it power and strength rather than reflecting God's loving image into the world.

Day 62

So let me tell you: don't worry about your life.
—Matthew 6:25

Brainy Tip: Worry and fear can cause neurochemical chaos in the brain and impact your mental and physical wellbeing.

We can only truly focus on one thing at a time. Multitasking is a myth; we can in theory do many things at once, but we will not do any of these things well. The same can be said of what we choose to think about. If we choose to focus on our fears and concerns, we allow them to take over our minds, shaping our future thoughts, words, and actions. And worrying almost never changes a situation!

God is bigger than any of our problems—he has got us covered! When we learn to trust in him, we can focus on what really matters: bringing heaven to earth through the way we live our lives. We can reflect his glory in everything we think, say, and do. We can focus on what can go right rather than what is going wrong. We should not run away from our problems, but we also should not let them control us.

Day 63

Therefore, my dear people, run away from idolatry.—1 Corinthians 10:14

> **Brainy Tip:** Whatever you love the most directs what you think, say, and do.

Sin—that is, a toxic mindset or worldview—starts with a thought. We focus our attention on something, thinking about it daily, giving it power and strength in the substrates of our brain through the quantum signals we send. We essentially make it our idol: our attention is worship.

In the writings of the apostle Paul, sin begins with idolatry.[1] We don't just do something bad out of the blue. Wrongdoing always starts in the mind, and as we think about it, allowing it to shape what we say and do, we trade in the image of God for an idol, whether it is bitterness, jealousy, power, sex, money, or anything other than God, who is love. We become what we think about the most, so we need to constantly be aware of what we are thinking. If you have a toxic pattern that is manifesting in your life, this means you have dedicated time to growing it over sixty-three-plus days—the time it takes to build a good, or a bad, habit.

Day 64

From that time on Jesus began to make his proclamation. "Repent!" he would say. "The kingdom of heaven is arriving!"—Matthew 4:17

Brainy Tip: Regardless of what has happened in the past, the brain can change. This process is called neuroplasticity.

In the Greek New Testament, repentance means to "change one's mind."[1] Toxic thinking creates idols, which lead to sin, or missing the mark of being a human made in God's image. If sin starts with our thinking, it needs to end with our thinking: a renewed mind is the key to true repentance and change.

With the help of the Holy Spirit we can take our thoughts captive and change the way we think, hence changing the way we speak and act. We can truly begin to offer ourselves up as God's servants, reflecting his glory and bringing heaven to earth. When we change the way we think, "the kingdom of heaven" can truly arrive!

Day 65

The steadfast love of the LORD never ceases, his mercies never come to an end; they are new every morning; great is your faithfulness.—Lamentations 3:22–23

Brainy Tip: If you wire it in, you can wire it out!

Many of us have had periods in our lives when we feel that we do not deserve to be saved. How could God ever forgive us? Can we ever change? Will things ever get better?

The good news is *yes*! Regardless of what has happened in the past, regardless of what has happened today, you can change. Through directed attention and effort, you can wire toxic thoughts out of your brain, replacing them with healthy, wired-for-love thoughts that allow you to reflect God's glory into the world. Your mind is separate from your brain but works through it, so they are integrally interconnected. With your mind, you change your brain. If you have wired it in, you can wire it out!

Day 66

In all these things we are completely victorious through the one who loved us.—Romans 8:37

> **Brainy Tip:** Our ability to think, feel, and choose is incredibly powerful!

Our ability to think is incredibly powerful—a gift from a loving, generous God. It can determine the way we speak and act, and it can determine the way we interact with the world around us. Even if we have failed time and time again, we can still change: as long as we live, our minds can change our brains through our thoughts. As long as we have breath, the structure of our brains can change and we can grow new brain cells, allowing us to achieve peak happiness, thinking, and health. This truly is the love of the Messiah! We are victorious when we choose to operate in his unconditional, perfect love.

Day 67

Jesus looked around at them. "Humanly speaking," he replied, "it's impossible. But everything's possible with God."
—Matthew 19:26

Brainy Tip: It is never too late to change your thinking.

Have you ever been told you cannot change? That you are what you are? Have you ever felt that your life will never get better? Do you feel stuck in a rut, lost, or helpless?

Change is always possible. Not only is it possible but it is happening all day long as you think—and you direct that change! Regardless of where you are, where you have been, or even where you will be, you can change your thinking *in the right direction* with the help of the Holy Spirit. You can change your mind, renewing it on a daily basis and taking your thoughts captive. And by changing your mind, you can change your life. You change the way you see and interact with the world, bringing heaven to earth through what you think, say, and do. This change is not only possible but a necessary part of life.

Day 68

This, you see, is how much God loved the world: enough to give his only, special son, so that everyone who believes in him should not be lost but should share in the life of God's new age.—John 3:16

> **Brainy Tip:** When we change the way we think, we change the way we live our lives.

God loves the entire world; he was willing to sacrifice his own Son so that all of creation could be made new again, so that we can *all* "share in the life to come." And this renewal process starts in our minds; when we change the way we think, we change the way we live our lives.

By taking our thoughts captive, by allowing the Holy Spirit to shape what we think, say, and do, we can begin to share in God's new life in the present. We can live fully in the "now" moments. We can turn the regrets into victories; we can turn the if-onlys into new ideas; we can turn our mistakes into positive learning experiences.

Day 69

For surely I know the plans I have for you, says the LORD, *plans for your welfare and not for harm, to give you a future with hope.*—Jeremiah 29:11

Brainy Tip: Hope is essential for mental and physical wellbeing. Quantum physics shows that the world is filled with possibilities that can give us hope for the future.

We live in a world where a million and one things can go wrong. We can get hurt, and often it is not hard to lose hope. It can be difficult to believe things will get better. We have all been there!

Yet when we trust in God's good plan for our lives, when we believe that, regardless of our circumstances, we have a "future with hope," we can begin to live out that hope in the present. Gratitude, love, and hope change our brains and bodies for the better because we are wired for love—we are made in the image of God, who is love.

Indeed, we live in a world filled with the ingredients of all our hopes and dreams. We become more well equipped to face the challenges of life when we trust in God's perfect plan for our lives and have hope for the future.

Day 70

O give thanks to the God of heaven, for his steadfast love endures forever.—Psalm 136:26

Brainy Tip: Love is incredibly powerful. It can heal the brain and body, allowing us to function at our best as we live our lives.

Regardless of where you are in your life, you can rely on God's love. You can trust in his faithfulness. When you allow yourself to be consumed by his love, you can allow this love to transform your mind, brain, and body for the better. You can be an example of his love in the world.

You can reflect his glory into creation in your unique and wonderful way, because your healthy mind and brain will generate love-filled quantum energy in a unique way when you choose to operate in love. People will literally feel the love coming out of you!

Day 71

I am persuaded, you see, that neither death nor life, nor angels nor rulers, nor the present, nor the future, nor powers, nor height, nor depth, nor any other creature will be able to separate us from the love of God in King Jesus our Lord.
—Romans 8:38–39

Brainy Tip: We are wired for love; we are designed to act, and react, in love.

We are wired to think, speak, and act in love. Nothing can separate us from the love that forms the core of our existence, God's love, unless we choose to reject his love.

When we get an insight into this love, we allow God's love to rule our lives, renewing our minds on a daily basis, and then we can reflect this beautiful love into the world. We can bring the culture of heaven to earth, participating in King Jesus's restoration project for the whole of creation. We can be victorious in our efforts to change ourselves, our communities, and our world for the better.

All of this starts with understanding what this love feels like, and we can do this by thinking about our loved ones and how they make us feel, watching a beautiful movie, playing with our pets, having a deep conversation with a close friend, watching the wind rustle through the trees on a beautiful day, or helping someone in need. If we are faithful with the small, everyday things, we will experience God's love in every area of our lives—we will experience the glory of God in the "now" moments of our life. We will see how God never leaves us. His love is ever-present, unconditional, and enduring.

Day 72

Don't owe anything to anyone, except the debt of mutual love. If you love your neighbor, you see, you have fulfilled the law.—Romans 13:8

Brainy Tip: When we treat others with love and respect, we positively influence our own health.

When we treat others with respect and love, we impact not only their lives but also our own. True, unconditional love has the power to positively influence the way our minds, brains, and bodies function, allowing us to become the best versions of ourselves that we can be. This love in turn helps us face the challenges of life.

When we experience love and when we give love, we give ourselves and others the courage to face adversity and suffering. It makes us *all* stronger and more resilient. We still experience the vagaries of life, but we do not let them determine how we treat ourselves or how we treat others!

We can love no matter what comes our way.

Day 73

Every person should be quick to hear, slow to speak, slow to anger.—James 1:19

> **Brainy Tip:** Bitterness, resentment, and anger negatively impact our physical and mental health.

When we do not treat others with respect and love, we negatively impact our own health. Rage, resentment, offense, bitterness, and jealousy, to name just several unsavory emotions, release toxic chemicals in the brain and body that can, over time, severely affect the quality of our lives. They create neurochemical chaos in the brain and body!

We should always try to act in love and forgiveness. We should be slow to anger and slow to react. By watching what we think and say about other people, and how we act toward others, we can positively influence our health and the health of our communities—we can truly be a light in the world.

Day 74

Whatever you want people to do to you, do that to them.
—Luke 6:31

> **Brainy Tip:** How you treat others will affect how you treat yourself.

We all have bad days, days where everyone and everything seems to get on our nerves and we have no qualms telling people exactly how irritating they are. It is almost as if there is a dark cloud over our heads as we go about our day, and people seem to part like the Red Sea before us.

Negative attitudes, just like positive attitudes, are contagious. We are all connected; in quantum physics, this is known as the principle of entanglement. We are entangled in each other's lives. The way we treat others, therefore, will both directly and indirectly affect the way we treat ourselves—if we put bad in, we get bad out. Our thoughts, words, and actions do not exist in a vacuum.

You cannot hide a bad attitude, but you can take it captive and change the way you think, speak, and act, reflecting God's love into the world rather than your own anger and frustration.

Day 75

A generous person will be enriched, and one who gives water will get water.—Proverbs 11:25

Brainy Tip: The more you think about loving others, the more you will love others.

The more we think about how we can love others, the more we are generous with our love, and the more we will act and speak in love. The more we act, and react, in love, the more we will change our world for the better. We can create communities that truly care for and support people.

Rather than sitting back, complaining how bad the world is, and waiting for Jesus to return, we should create communities that nourish everyone, including ourselves, and help us all bring heaven to earth through our thoughts, words, and actions. The desire for a better world starts with us, so start spreading that love today!

Day 76

Children, let us not love in word, or in speech, but in deed and in truth.—1 John 3:18

> **Brainy Tip:** If you think good thoughts, you will say and do good things.

Like athletes training for a competition, we need to train ourselves to think, speak, and act like the Messiah. We have to train the muscles of our minds, so that when we find ourselves in challenging situations we can speak and act in love.

Character development doesn't happen overnight. If we want to truly love other people, we need to build that love into our minds. We need to go way beyond positive affirmations and superficial, empty "I love yous" and genuinely begin to care for people "in deed and in truth." It is important to mean what we say and do; otherwise we create cognitive dissonance in our minds, which leads to damage in our brains and bodies. Being at war with ourselves is never a good idea.

Day 77

So, now, faith, hope, and love remain, these three; and, of them, love is the greatest.—1 Corinthians 13:13

Brainy Tip: If you think love, you will act in love.

If God is love, the more we think, speak, and act in love, the more we experience God—the more we see his face. When we build habits of loving others into our brains through our choices, we develop a worldview that is based on true love, the kind of love the apostle Paul spoke about in both of his letters to the Corinthians. This worldview will shape our future words and actions, allowing us to bring heaven to earth as we interact with the world around us.

Make the guidelines in 1 Corinthians 13 part of your mental self-care regimen. Train yourself to speak and act with patience and kindness; stop all envy and jealousy of others; stop demanding your own way; stop keeping a record of wrongs; do not ignore or rejoice when you see injustice being done; celebrate when truth wins; never give up, never lose hope, and endure through even the most difficult of times!

Day 78

Blessings on the pure in heart! You will see God.—Matthew 5:8

Brainy Tip: Love transforms us spiritually, mentally, and physically by literally changing brain chemistry, quantum energy, and genetic expression!

It seems like everyone is always looking for a simple solution to their problems. So many people ask me how they can change their thinking, but few actually want to work hard at changing.

Although real love is not necessarily quick or simple or easy, it is a solution to many problems—if not all. When we begin to genuinely love others, we experience God, who is love. The divine is infused throughout our everyday existence, transforming us and everyone and everything around us. It has the power to make us "pure of heart." Love, as the source of all existence, is the most powerful force in the universe; it truly can change the world.

Day 79

Love must be real. Hate what is evil; stick fast to what is good.—Romans 12:9

Brainy Tip: What you allow into your mind will create your unique reality and determine the way you live your life.

If we are constantly angry, bitter, jealous, and envious, our brains become toxic. Not only does this increase our chance of getting physically ill but we also cannot genuinely love others, even if we are still nice to people or do something good for someone.

"Love must be real." Unless we change the way we think about people, renewing our minds and developing a worldview that is based on love, we cannot genuinely care for other people and will find it difficult to "stick fast to what is good." We will keep failing, because we never really tried to build a habit of love into our brains in the first place.

Day 80

Anyone who doesn't love abides in death.—1 John 3:14

Brainy Tip: Hating others negatively impacts our health.

As God is the source of all existence, and God is love, when we do not think, act, and speak in love we bring death and destruction into the world. When we *choose* to respond negatively to our circumstances and when we *choose* to respond in uncontrolled anger and hatred, we negatively impact not only our relationships but also our mental and physical health.

Many studies highlight the connection between hatred and mental and physical illness. Hatred and bitterness have actually been shown to reduce life expectancy and set people up for many diseases, including heart disease and cancer!

None of us can afford to hate others, because we will bring death into our lives.

Day 81

"Be angry, but don't sin"; don't let the sun go down on you while you're angry.—Ephesians 4:26

Brainy Tip: The more you think toxic thoughts, the more power you give these thoughts over your life and the more damage you do to your brain and body.

There will be times in your life when anger is the most appropriate response to an unfair or dangerous situation. For example, if your child is trying to touch a hot stove, if your friend is running across a busy street without looking either way for oncoming traffic, or if someone you love is abused, you should get angry at the threat to the sanctity of human life.

But when does anger become a sin? How does uncontrolled or uncalled-for anger affect our humanity? When you think about a situation and how angry it made you feel *over time*, allowing the "sun to go down" on your feelings, you build a negative mindset into your brain, giving it the power to shape your thoughts, words, and actions in the future. You allow it to grow, and, like weeds in a flower bed, its bitterness can spread and affect the way you live your life, your health included. It is therefore incredibly important that you do not allow negative feelings like anger or bitterness to fester. If you are angry with someone, deal with the situation. Do not give this anger the power to affect the quality of your life.

Day 82

But now you must put away the lot of them: anger, rage, wickedness, blasphemy, dirty talk coming out of your mouth.
—Colossians 3:8

Brainy Tip: What you say is based on what you think.

Words are never just words. Even if they feel impulsive, they are based on thoughts you have built inside your head through your choices. What we say, like what we do, is a reflection of how we think—our mindsets shape our words. What we choose to think about will pour out into our lives.

We should therefore keep a close eye on what we choose to say to people, because it is an indication of what is going on inside our heads. If we find ourselves falling into a spiral of "dirty talk," we should stop ourselves and work on renewing our minds before this toxicity has time to affect our mental and physical health. We should make sure that our thoughts, words, and actions are life-giving.

Day 83

Where do wars come from? Why do people among you fight?
It all comes from within, doesn't it.—James 4:1

Brainy Tip: Everything you say and do is first a thought.

If you want to make a good meal, you need good-quality ingredients. It is a matter of "what goes in comes out." It goes without saying that you cannot make a delicious dinner with rotten ingredients.

The same is true with our thinking. If we want to see a better world, we have to change the way we think (good in, good out), because our thoughts are the root of what we say and do. Everything good—but also everything bad—comes from "within." If we renew our minds and change the way we think, we can change our lives. The power of our thoughts cannot be underestimated!

Day 84

Keep your heart with all vigilance, for from it flow the springs of life.—Proverbs 4:23

> **Brainy Tip:** What we think has the power to bring life or death into our brains, our bodies, and the world.

Thoughts are real things that impact brain, mind, and body functionality. If you do not capture your thoughts and monitor incoming information, negative thoughts can take root, which can steal your mental peace, affect your ability to build useful memory and learn, and make you ill; toxic thoughts can bring forth death. Your thinking will become foggy, you will lack wisdom, and your memory will be affected.

If, however, you allow healthy, love-based thoughts to take root in your mind, you can bring forth the "springs of life." You will improve your mental and physical health, which will allow you to truly be a light in the world, reflecting God's majestic love and glory.

Day 85

So fasten your belts—the belts of your minds! Keep yourselves under control. Set your hope completely on the grace that will be given you when Jesus the Messiah is revealed.—1 Peter 1:13

Brainy Tip: Controlling your thoughts is a lifestyle, not a task.

Remember, thoughts are real structures inside your brain, structures that grow and become stronger the more you think about something. As you think, you activate genetic expression and make proteins, which hold your thoughts. Our memories are stored in these minute quantum neuro-biological computers.

When you choose to focus on something, you give it quantum energy and, therefore, power. If it is positive, it can enhance your mental and physical health. If it is negative, it can negatively impact your health, especially if you think about it over time—you essentially give this thought power over your life.

What you think about will determine your behavior, so you need to control your mind on a daily basis if you want to "keep yourself under control." Mental issues are not pre-programmed diseases of the brain; they are toxic thoughts that have been allowed to run amok inside your brain. You need to focus on God's love and grace and the example of the Messiah every day, because the more you think about reflecting his glory, the more you *will* reflect his glory, thereby revealing his love to a broken world.

Day 86

"What makes someone unclean," [Jesus] went on, "is what comes out of them. Evil intentions come from inside, out of people's hearts."—Mark 7:20–21

Brainy Tip: Your behavior reflects your mindset.

You cannot hide your thoughts, even if you feel you can. What you think affects what you say, what you do, and what you think in the future! What is inside your mind, what you think about and pay attention to the most, will eventually bubble up to the surface and overflow in your life.

How? When you pay attention to something, it is converted to physical matter in your brain, changing the structure of your little quantum neurobiological computers. Toxic thinking damages these, which are delicate and designed to hold only healthy thoughts. Consequently, whatever is inside these structures will emerge as words and actions in your life if they are strengthened with continual thinking. What you think about the most, your mindset, directly affects your behavior.

When your thought life is toxic, it can make your behavior "unclean." It can hurt your relationships and your mental and physical health. You should therefore constantly watch what you think; you should never stop examining what is in your "heart" or inner person. Who are you at your core? Who have you become? What do your thoughts say about you as a person?

Day 87

We have all become like one who is unclean, and all our righteous deeds are like a filthy cloth. We all fade like a leaf, and our iniquities, like the wind, take us away.—Isaiah 64:6

Brainy Tip: You cannot hide bad thinking habits.

Our thinking shapes and colors everything we say and do. We merge with our environments, so whatever we focus on will become realities in our lives. If we have bad thinking habits, such as jealousy, hatred, and bitterness, we will speak and act in a negative manner, notwithstanding our "righteous deeds."

We may think we are getting away with thinking a bad thought about someone by saying nice things to their face or doing something nice for them; however, unless our words and actions match what is in our hearts (that is, in our minds), we will cause chaos and confusion in our brains and bodies, which will impact our ability to function in life.

We need to deal with our toxic thoughts, not hide them under the carpet, because at some point these thoughts will burst out, and we will say or do something that reflects how we *really* feel. This discrepancy between what we really think and what we say is called cognitive dissonance and is toxic to our health, potentially decreasing our life expectancy—bad thinking can make us essentially "fade like leaves."

Day 88

The beginning of strife is like letting out water; so stop before the quarrel breaks out.—Proverbs 17:14

Brainy Tip: If you control your thinking, you can control your reactions to the circumstances of life.

By standing outside yourself and observing your own thinking, you can take your thoughts captive and renew your mind. Your frontal lobe will fire up in response to your decision to observe your thinking—I call this the multiple perspective advantage (MPA), which enables you to stop yourself before you say those words, do that thing, or react in that way.

Because of the wonderful way God designed your brain, you are more than capable of stopping a negative situation from spiraling out of control. You can stop the water from flowing before the barrel breaks—before your thinking gets you into trouble. You don't have to live your life like a hot mess!

Day 89

When the cares of my heart are many, your consolations cheer my soul.—Psalm 94:19

> **Brainy Tip:** We can choose how we react to hard times by choosing what we focus on during hard times.

There will be times in your life when you feel bombarded by a million and one problems. It is almost as if you are drowning in anxiety and can barely breathe. We have all been there. We all know what it feels like to be overwhelmed by life's cares.

Yet we do not have to let these cares overcome us. We do not have to be a victim of our circumstances, even when the "cares of our hearts" are many. By *choosing* to focus on God's love and strength during challenging times, we can find the inner strength to face whatever life throws our way. Not only is this possible but we are designed to do this!

We do not have to be pushed around by our circumstances. We can find joy even amid great sadness. We can feel pain and yet know that there is hope for victory. We can be consoled in the knowledge of God's tender grace and care, because we know that God is the ultimate source of all reality.

Day 90

Do not fear, for I am with you, do not be afraid, for I am your God; I will strengthen you, I will help you, I will uphold you with my victorious right hand.—Isaiah 41:10

> **Brainy Tip:** The mind works through the brain and therefore controls the brain, so you can be victorious over your biology and your circumstances.

There will be many times in your life when you feel like giving up. There will be times when you will curl up in a ball, cry, and wish it all would end. Life is not easy but it can still be beautiful—even amid all the pain, suffering, and heartache.

Human beings are incredibly resilient and incredibly powerful—you are incredibly resilient and incredibly powerful! When you learn to recognize the power in your mind, trusting in God's grace and his strength in you, you will recognize that *impossible* is a word, not a life sentence. You do not have to fear what can happen or has happened. You are you, and that is enough because you are made in the image of the Most High God. Never forget that the essence of who you are is the pure and wonderful power of love.

Day 91

I have strength for everything in the one who gives me power.—Philippians 4:13

> **Brainy Tip:** The brain is the substrate through which the mind works—it reflects the action of the mind. The mind controls the brain; the brain does not control the mind.

No matter what you have faced, are facing, or will face, you have an *incredible* mind and brain that were created by an *incredible* God. Your mind has the power to change the direction of your life and create new and exciting realities, even if the world puts a thousand roadblocks in your way. Remember: the mind controls the brain. Your mind controls the physical direction of your life. You really can do all things through the Messiah, because in him you have the power of the universe behind you; you have the power of love inside you.

Day 92

This is the day that the LORD has made; let us rejoice and be glad in it.—Psalm 118:24

Brainy Tip: Our choices determine how we respond to our environment, and our brain reflects our responses.

Focusing on the positive allows you to see multiple possibilities in every situation. This type of thinking is intrinsically hopeful; you just keep on trying till you find success. You are grateful for the journey *and* the destination. And the good news is that this is part of the wired-for-love nature of the brain and body—you just have to unlock it!

Research on the effects gratitude has on our biology shows how being thankful increases our longevity, our ability to use our imagination, our ability to solve problems, and our overall health. Gratitude for where we are is essential for where we want to be.

Look at Thomas Edison. He tried about a thousand times before he succeeded in inventing the light bulb. When asked about his "failures," Edison declared that "I have gotten lots of results! I know several thousand things that won't work!'"[1] Edison didn't limit his potential to preconceived notions of success. He had a goal and he kept going until he achieved it, regardless of the number of attempts along the way. He didn't see his attempts as failures; he saw his attempts as *results*. He had *gained worthwhile knowledge*—it was a learning process. The question is, what have you gained from your life experiences?

Day 93

But you, take courage! Do not let your hands be weak, for your work shall be rewarded.—2 Chronicles 15:7

> **Brainy Tip:** Hard work increases your intelligence and improves your health.

The ability to think is truly phenomenal. Our brains can change as we think (neuroplasticity) and grow new brain cells (neurogenesis). Using the incredible power in our minds, we can persist and grow in response to life's challenges. Frequent, positive, and challenging learning experiences can actually increase intelligence in a relatively short amount of time! So do not let your work get the better of you. Remember that the power inside you is greater than anything that comes your way, and if you persist you will be rewarded, mentally and physically. You are as intelligent as you want to be!

Day 94

Whatever you do, give it your very best, as if you were working for the master [God] and not for human beings.
—Colossians 3:23

Brainy Tip: Persistence and discipline are essential to mental and physical wellbeing.

We all have times in our lives when we just feel like being "Netflix and chill" lazy. I mean, do we really have to do that task? Do we really have to write that paper? Do we really have to clean that kitchen? Let's face it: we don't always want to "give our very best," especially when a new season of our favorite TV show is available!

Yet our minds and brains are designed to thrive when we push through and try our best. The harder we work, the more disciplined we are in completing a task, the more our brain grows in a positive direction and the more our intelligence increases, improving the health of not only our brains but also our bodies. We should treat every task we are faced with as a gift from God to help us grow and develop as human beings, even if we don't necessarily get it right the first time. Failure is not the end of the world—it is the beginning of new growth in the brain. Indolence and giving up, however, can negatively impact our mental and physical wellbeing.

Day 95

In all toil there is profit, but mere talk leads only to poverty.—Proverbs 14:23

Brainy Tip: Words alone do not lead to success.

It is wonderful to make plans, have ideas, and write out your goals. Yet there comes a time when talk is not enough; there comes a time when good, honest, hard work is necessary for your dreams to become realities. You can create realities with your thinking, which impacts what you say and do, but to build these realities in your head and life requires effort over time—you have to think and do. As the saying goes, Rome wasn't built in a day!

Day 96

But be people who do the word, not merely people who hear it and deceive themselves.—James 1:22

Brainy Tip: Positive affirmations need to be supported by congruent positive beliefs.

Your words have to be backed up with honesty and integrity, or what in psychological terms is called cognitive congruence. Positive affirmations only work when you believe what you say—the root and the fruit need to match. If you lie to yourself, you will experience cognitive dissonance, the opposite of cognitive congruence, which can impact your mental and physical health because you are creating an internal war between what you actually believe and what you want to believe. You can quote as many Bible verses as you want to yourself, but unless you believe what they say, implanting the Word deep into your mind, you will not be able to follow the Messiah in thought, word, and deed.

Day 97

The mouths of the righteous utter wisdom, and their tongues speak justice. The law of their God is in their hearts; their steps do not slip.—Psalm 37:30–31

Brainy Tip: An examined life is a life that produces wisdom. So, as you choose to deliberately live a self-regulated and disciplined thought life, you will have an organized and healthy brain.

Good words, words that are wise and speak of justice, come from what we have planted inside our mind, our "hearts." As you choose to deliberately live a self-regulated and disciplined thought life, you will have an organized and healthy brain that allows you to make wise decisions.

We are constantly building memories and updating our nonconscious mind with new information and increased levels of expertise and wisdom—if we choose correctly and think about things that bring life and hope. If we choose incorrectly, however, our updated memory and knowledge are toxic and brain-damaging. These toxic memory networks impact what we say, what we do, our overall wellbeing, and our relationships. Both wisdom and foolishness come from within; it is up to us what we choose to build into our brains and live out in our lives.

Day 98

A gentle tongue is a tree of life, but perverseness in it breaks the spirit.—Proverbs 15:4

Brainy Tip: Your words are important. They reflect what you are thinking, choosing, and feeling.

The words you speak are electromagnetic and quantum life forces that come from thoughts inside your brain, which you build into your mind by thinking, feeling, and choosing over time. These words contain power and reflect your thought life, influencing the world around you and the circumstances of your life. Your words are therefore very useful, since they provide insight into what is holding you back, breaking your spirit, or propelling you forward—your "tree of life."

Day 99

If anyone supposes that they are devout, and does not control their tongue, but rather deceives their heart—such a person's devotion is futile.—James 1:26

Brainy Tip: You speak what you think.

The words you speak feed back into the physical thoughts you have built into your mind, reinforcing the memory they came from. When you make negative statements and are not "controlling your tongue," you release negative chemicals. These negative memories grow stronger the more you think about them and speak about them, and become negative strongholds that control your attitude and life. Words can "deceive your heart."

Day 100

My dear family, when you find yourselves tumbling into various trials and tribulations, learn to look at it with complete joy.—James 1:2

Brainy Tip: Your perceptions are based on how you choose to see things.

We all have to face our own mountains, our own demons, and our own skeletons in the closet. None of us are issue-free. We all have "trials and tribulations" we have to face. Nevertheless, we cannot use our circumstances as excuses not to succeed in life. A victim mentality will get us nowhere.

Being able to see possibilities and experience a deep sense of joy and hope in the midst of your difficulties is a *game-changer*. It transforms your thinking, allowing you to keep running your race. It is the key to success, even when you cannot see the end of the road. It is what gives you the power to move mountains and create miracles in your life.

Day 101

We also celebrate in our sufferings, because we know that suffering produces patience, patience produces a well-formed character, and a character like that produces hope.—Romans 5:3–4

> **Brainy Tip:** Challenges strengthen our minds, and because the mind works through the brain, a strong mind means a strong brain.

Challenges can bring out the best in us and heal our brains, depending on our reaction to what we are going through. Choosing to get to the other side of a challenge brings a sense of happiness in the achievement and sets the stage for the next challenge with the addition of new skills gained. The strength of character that we build through this is reflected in the circuitry of the brain and helps to sustain us in the future.

We need to choose to be happy, push through our challenges, and enjoy the process of developing our abilities. If we fail, we need to pick ourselves up, even if we don't feel like it, because great things are happening in our brain! Despite how we initially feel, choosing to be happy will become the energy source that keeps us going.

Day 102

Celebrate your hope; be patient in suffering; give constant energy to prayer.—Romans 12:12

Brainy Tip: Happiness is an internal state of mind.

We are not merely happy or unhappy. Our happiness does not depend on our circumstances. As Harvard professor Shawn Achor notes, "it's a cultural myth that we cannot change our happiness."[1] A positive, love-based mindset and an ability to make a stressful situation work for us are completely under our control. Instead of freaking out when things do not go as hoped or planned, we can choose to "freak out in the love zone," as I mentioned on day 47. We can get upset or angry, but we give our feelings over to God in prayer, reminding ourselves that God's strength is in us and that we have the necessary inner resources to cope and to conquer.

Day 103

Beloved, do not believe every spirit. Rather, test the spirits to see whether they are from God.—1 John 4:1

Brainy Tip: Expectations can lead to realities.

Many times it feels like there is a tiny voice inside our heads, telling us that something is going to fail, that we are not good enough to do something, or that we will never get it right because we have failed so many times in the past. Don't choose to listen to that voice! Don't let those words shape your expectations for the future.

It is important to understand that our expectations change the structure of our brain. Learned associations result in *real* physiological and cognitive outcomes. If these associations are positive, they are known as the placebo effect. In essence, when we learn to expect good things, good things start to happen, such as more energy, improved immune function, and better mental and physical performance. Yet the opposite is also true; thinking bad things are going to happen often allows bad things to happen—this is known as the nocebo effect!

Fear is real and can build negative learned associations in the brain that affect our future thoughts, words, and actions. Bad expectations can create bad realities, but they don't have to! Do not let your past or your present fears determine your future. Use your powerful imagination to change the way you see your future. This is not just a simple law of attraction or wishful thinking. When your expectations match your beliefs and goals and align with God's love, you can do the impossible and change the world for the better.

Day 104

Enter his gates with thanksgiving, and his courts with praise.
Give thanks to him, bless his name.—Psalm 100:4

Brainy Tip: Gratitude improves mental and physical health.

When we choose to be grateful, we tap into our natural design. Research on the effects gratitude has on our biology shows how being thankful increases our longevity, our ability to use our imagination, our ability to problem-solve, and our overall health.

Counting your blessings now actually makes it easier to recognize them later because your mind will get better and better at the process of building a positive and grateful mindset, so start making this part of your daily mental self-care routine. If you train your mind to see the glass as half full, it will soon be overflowing!

Day 105

The LORD is my strength and my shield; in him my heart trusts; so I am helped, and my heart exults, and with my song I give thanks to him.—Psalm 28:7

Brainy Tip: You are as happy as you want to be; happiness is a choice. The happier you are, the healthier your brain is.

Life is tough, but it can also be beautiful. Happiness, satisfaction, and success are not static markers in a linear life; they are as dynamic and powerful as your thinking makes them, regardless of your circumstances. You can be in the ugliest place in the world, with a million deadlines and the uncertainty of tomorrow, and you can still smile and laugh and enjoy the "now" moment.

The knowledge that God is behind you, that he is your "strength and shield," gives you hope and the courage to smile every moment of every day. His love and care are always present; God is always faithful. Nothing can separate you from his love, a love that wants you to succeed and live up to your full potential.

Day 106

Don't let your hearts be troubled; don't be fearful.—John 14:27

Brainy Tip: Positively responding to stress can positively affect your mental and physical health.

Like everything in life, the way you view stressful situations can affect the way you deal with tough situations. This is liberating because research shows that the way you view stress can make your body work for you or against you! Depending on *your* perceptions, you can make a difficult situation work for you or against you. You are not helpless; you have the power to change your reality.

If you face a difficult situation with a "glass half full" instead of a "glass half empty" attitude, not allowing your heart to "be troubled," the blood vessels around your heart begin to dilate. Increased blood flow results in increased oxygen flowing to your brain, which, in turn, increases your cognitive fluency and clarity of thought—that is, your ability to not only face a challenge but overcome it. This increased blood flow also balances the sympathetic and parasympathetic nervous systems, fueling intellectual growth. A genetic switch will be turned on inside the hippocampus of your brain, which strengthens your body, allowing you to cope in a difficult situation. More than fourteen hundred neurophysiological responses will be activated, allowing you to stay strong amid adversity.

Day 107

The way to keep your lives is to be patient.—Luke 21:19

Brainy Tip: Stress can work for or against you.

When you read about the negative health effects of not managing stress correctly, you can get stressed out about being stressed out, which allows all those negative consequences to negatively affect you. It is like when you read about the dangers of not sleeping and how bad it is for you and then you cannot sleep because you are worrying about not sleeping. (We have all been there!) Often there is so much emphasis on what is bad for us and what can go wrong that we forget to focus on what is good for us.

Being patient with our circumstances and strong amid challenges, relying on the future hope we have in Jesus the Messiah, and realizing that we can make our bodies work for us or against us just by our perceptions enables us to push through difficult times, thereby "keeping our lives." We do not have to let stress get the better of us and ruin our health and our lives. Remember, our perception of stress is key and is under *our* control. We can face whatever comes our way, and we can deal with it.

It is all a matter of perspective.

Day 108

Are you having a real struggle? Come to me! Are you carrying a big load on your back? Come to me—I'll give you a rest!—Matthew 11:28

Brainy Tip: We have, within the design of our genome, a genetic switch that is activated when we perceive stress in a positive light, which increases our resilience in stressful situations.

The Scriptures do not promise that we will never face hard times. They do, however, constantly remind us that God is always with us. He never leaves our side; he is a place of rest and refuge.

Indeed, we can have confidence in the way he has designed our minds and brains. For example, within the design of our genome is a genetic switch that is activated when we perceive stress as positive, which increases our resilience in stressful situations. How amazing is our God!

There are times we may feel we don't have any power over our lives or circumstances, but we do! Our ability to think, feel, and choose is innately powerful and resilient—we have minds that are more potent than all the smartphones on the planet *combined*. We are more than equipped to deal with whatever comes our way.

Day 109

For it was you who formed my inward parts; you knit me together in my mother's womb.—Psalm 139:13

> **Brainy Tip:** The law of the brain is diversity, which means the thoughts you build into your brain are completely unique to you. No one thinks, speaks, or acts like you do.

A large part of not being able to deal with stress in a positive manner comes with low self-esteem and a lack of confidence in your abilities. It is important to remember that you are amazing. You can do something no one else can do. You can think like no one else can—this is known as the law of diversity in the brain. You were created and designed by an incredible God to do incredible things. You have something great to give to the world. Why settle for less when you are so much more?

Take the time to truly believe in yourself. If you don't have confidence in your abilities, no matter how skilled and talented you are, your performance and health will suffer.

Day 110

Your hands have made and fashioned me.—Psalm 119:73

Brainy Tip: What *you* think matters.

Every thought you think matters because it changes your brain. You create your unique reality and shape your brain with your unique thoughts. You have been designed by God with a beautiful way of thinking, specific to you and evident from infancy. No one thinks like you; no one will ever think like you. There is something you can do that no one else can do.

The more you discover how you uniquely think, feel, and choose, the more you will understand the blueprint of your incredible identity, your purpose, and your part in the kingdom as a child of the Most High God. The more you discover who you are at your core, the more you will love the person you were created to be.

Day 111

Before I formed you in the womb I knew you.—Jeremiah 1:5

Brainy Tip: You are the only one who can do what you can do, because your mind activates your brain in a way that is different from every other person on the planet.

God doesn't make mistakes. He created you with intention and purpose. If you find yourself in a bad place in life, remember that this is not who you are at your core but rather who you have become. You can change. You can find yourself, your "youness," again.

Although you may not think you do, you actually know who you are! Your identity flows out of how you think, speak, and act, and the more you recognize how wonderful your true identity is, the more you can embrace this identity and bring heaven to earth in your unique way.

Remember, you are designed to reflect a unique part of the image of the divine. Your worth and dignity are intrinsically tied to God's magnificence. When you are you, we all get to know God better.

Day 112

We are the clay, and you are our potter; we are all the work of your hand.—Isaiah 64:8

Brainy Tip: You have a customized thinking pattern—your own customized mode of thinking.

Your Perfect You, the unique way God has shaped and crafted you, is like a filter or a screen. When this filter is locked up by low self-esteem or toxic thinking, you are not free to be you. We have all been there: we feel like there is a battle inside us, like who we have become is fighting who we know, deep down, we really are. When you step out of your Perfect You, you will be in conflict, and this will make you frustrated and unhappy. It will even temporarily reduce your intelligence and potentially lead to mental and physical ill health!

Where your mind goes, your brain and body follow. When you learn to focus on God, who is love, and what he says about you, you learn how to embrace your unique identity and discover who you truly are in him.

Day 113

God saw everything that he had made, and indeed, it was very good.—Genesis 1:31

> **Brainy Tip:** Science confirms you are not a mistake, because no two brains, from the structural level to the quantum level, are the same. There is no "normal"; there is only unique.

Operating in your unique way of thinking, feeling, and choosing, or what I call your Perfect You, is a way for you to celebrate who you are. In a world where we are often told that we are not worthy or do not live up to a particular standard, that we are not "normal," this celebration is critical!

Indeed, we cannot truly live for God or transform our societies if we hate what we see in the mirror. Your Perfect You is so deeply and intrinsically wired into the fabric of who you are that when you recognize it, you develop an intimate awareness of and desire to be yourself. You recognize that who you are is fundamentally *good* and that you have so much to give to the world.

Day 114

Well then, we have gifts that differ in accordance with the grace that has been given to us, and we must use them appropriately.—Romans 12:6

Brainy Tip: We all think, feel, and choose differently.

There is no one like you, which means there is something you can do that no one else can do. Because of the unique way you think, feel, and choose, your experience of life will enhance mine. We are made differently, and we are designed to work together. When you are not you, and when I am not me, we all miss out on knowing God better, because we each reflect his image in a unique and beautiful way!

Day 115

But the fruit of the spirit is love, joy, peace, great-hearted-ness, kindness, generosity, faithfulness, gentleness, self-control. There is no law that opposes things like that!
—Galatians 5:22–23

Brainy Tip: When you learn to embrace who you are, you can operate in positive ways.

Once you begin to understand your Perfect You and its structure, you can begin to walk in anticipation and freedom through life, rejoicing despite the circumstances. Your Perfect You sets you free to be who you are and to do what you love.

Operating in your Perfect You brings satisfaction and contentment. It reveals your innermost qualities, which are bound in love, joy, peace, great-heartedness, kindness, generosity, faithfulness, gentleness, and self-control, because you are made in the image of the triune God. You can love yourself and others because you recognize God in all people, you can find joy and peace regardless of your circumstances, you can be kind and generous and faithful with what God has entrusted to you, and you can realize that you are in control of what you think, say, and do.

Day 116

They swapped the glory of the immortal God for the likeness of the image of mortal humans—and of birds, animals, and reptiles.—Romans 1:23

> **Brainy Tip:** You cannot truly be satisfied being something or someone you were not created to be.

In our current society, it can become very confusing to find any stable identity, so it is critical that we begin to understand what it means to be made in God's image. Each of us needs to find our unique part of his image, because if we don't, the world will brand us. Remember, we will become whatever we focus on the most. The Israelites exchanged their glories (their Perfect You as image-bearers of God) for the image of the golden calf, and we too can lose ourselves trying to be what we are not called to be.

We become what we love, so we must learn to love our God by seeing his incredible piece of eternity inside us. Focusing on God will increase the authenticity of our Perfect You; nothing else will satisfy us. You make a lousy someone else, but you make a Perfect You.

Day 117

Good trees can't produce bad fruit, nor can bad ones produce good fruit!—Matthew 7:18

Brainy Tip: Acting against your true nature of love and your beliefs can affect your mental and physical health.

In order to sustain a consistent outlook and pattern in your life, your spirit, thoughts, feelings, choices, words, and actions must line up. When you say or do something your brain doesn't "believe in," it is unsustainable and can become toxic. These toxic thoughts can affect your mental and physical health, your relationships, and the overall quality of your life.

Cognitive dissonance cannot be hidden. Living a lie is a roadblock on the road to success and happiness and will prevent you from living up to your full potential.

Day 118

Every creation of God, you see, is good.—1 Timothy 4:4

Brainy Tip: You are designed to be *you*.

You can try as hard as you can to be something or someone other than how God has designed you, but this will create conflict in your mind and body. At your core you will always try to return to your natural inclination—your Perfect You. Comparing yourself to others, trying to live up to impossible standards, or acting and speaking according to what you think others want can damage your mental and physical health, preventing you from being truly happy and healthy in life. You move away from the "good" way God designed you, losing your sense of peace and authenticity.

Day 119

God has made us what we are. God has created us in King Jesus for the good works that he prepared, ahead of time, as the road we must travel. —Ephesians 2:10

> **Brainy Tip:** You can't be as successful as someone else. Your success is determined by your uniqueness.

We must remember that success, in terms of *shalom* and holistic, biblical prosperity, is not defined by a collection of assets, an accumulation of power, or cash in the bank. If that were the formula, there would be no cares for those in the highest tax brackets. Rather, success is living out God's purpose for our lives, using the Perfect You he has given us to transform our community, and, in doing so, bringing heaven to earth. As a result, every single one of us will be successful in different ways, because every single one of us can do something no one else can do. We all have different "roads" we must travel.

Day 120

Just as the body is one, and has many members, and all the members of the body, though they are many, are one body, so also is the Messiah.—1 Corinthians 12:12

Brainy Tip: We are made for community.

Relationships, of course, would not be relationships if we were all the same. Our differences shape and enhance our relationships. Although we could never understand the impact of our thoughts on everyone around us, since we cannot know everything, we can get a sense of our interconnectedness when a loved one is sad and our hearts ache, or if we watch the news and feel compassion for people going through incredibly difficult circumstances. We all collectively represent God's magnificent creation. He is the whole system and we are the parts in him. No one is better than anyone else. Like cells in the human body, we originate from one source but have different functions depending on who and where we are within a larger community.

Day 121

He supplies the growth that the whole body needs, linked as it is and held together by every joint which supports it, with each member doing its own proper work. Then the body builds itself up in love.—Ephesians 4:16

Brainy Tip: We are designed to serve and love each other.

We have something unique to give to the world. Our communities need us! In fact, our brains and bodies respond positively when we become active members in a community. For example, the mesolimbic dopamine system, a system linked to addiction, lights up when we give to others, giving us a deep sense of pleasure. We are essentially hardwired to serve others, because service aligns with our wired-for-love design!

Day 122

You must put on love, which ties everything together and makes it complete.—Colossians 3:14

Brainy Tip: Science shows that love can heal us.

There is a massive "unlearning" of negative toxic thoughts when we operate in love. We can unlearn negative fear—it is not a part of our innate natural functioning, our Perfect You. Recent neuroscientific research demonstrates that the chemicals the brain releases when we are operating in our Perfect You include oxytocin, which literally melts away negative toxic thought clusters so that rewiring of new, nontoxic circuits can happen. This chemical also flows when we trust, bond, and reach out to others. So choosing to operate in the default nature of love literally can wipe out fear!

Day 123

How very good and pleasant it is when kindred live together in unity!—Psalm 133:1

> **Brainy Tip:** Our minds, brains, and bodies thrive when we positively interact with other people.

Human beings are social animals. Whether we like having alone time or not, we all need community. In fact, engaging positively with people in our social support network correlates with a number of desirable physical and mental outcomes. Community involvement has been associated with mental health and cognitive resilience, reduction of chronic pain, lower blood pressure, and improved cardiovascular health. We are designed to thrive in community!

Day 124

*Turn to me and be gracious to me, for I am lonely and af-
flicted. Relieve the troubles of my heart, and bring me out
of my distress.—Psalm 25:16–17*

Brainy Tip: Loneliness can negatively affect both our mental and physical health.

Isolation can negatively affect our wellbeing. Loneliness actually increases the risk for premature mortality among all ages,
making it a growing public health hazard. No wonder social
isolation has been used as a type of punishment or torture!
We should take the danger posed by isolation seriously. We
should all work together to build loving and resilient communities where we live.

Day 125

The one who lives alone is self-indulgent, showing contempt for all who have sound judgment.—Proverbs 18:1

Brainy Tip: Fantasies should never become more important than reality.

The more removed we become from human connection, the more potential there is for us to turn to the fantasy world as a replacement for reality rather than using our imagination as a tool to create successful and satisfying lives. We all, to a certain extent, fantasize about how things could or should be, and this imagining often encourages us to pursue our dreams. Yet our imagination should not be divorced from real life; otherwise our fantasies can become more important to us than reality. When our fantasies get that important, they often lead to long-term social isolation, which can dramatically affect our health and reduce our lifespan.

Day 126

Let us, as well, stir up one another's minds to energetic effort in love and good works.—Hebrews 10:24

Brainy Tip: The more we reach out in love, the more our brain and body respond in a positive direction.

Loneliness by its very nature is not something we can fix by ourselves. We have to reach out to all age groups and all spheres of society to combat social isolation and improve mental and physical health. It is important to encourage social connectedness in every area of our lives. We need to develop a holistic community mindset if we want to succeed in life and if we want to help others succeed at life. We need to constantly discover new ways of becoming active members in our community, thinking, speaking, and acting in love wherever possible.

Day 127

The aim of this is for you all to be like-minded, sympathetic and loving to one another, tender-hearted and humble.—1 Peter 3:8

Brainy Tip: We increase our rate of healing when we reach out to help others in our times of distress.

Have you ever helped someone in need, or spent a day at a shelter or a soup kitchen? Nothing can ever replace the feeling of reaching out in love. These moments are priceless—moments when we can feel the presence of heaven on earth.

In fact, research shows that when we do good things and reach out in love, endorphins and serotonin are released that make us feel great. These chemicals detox our brains, heal us, and increase our motivation and wisdom, helping us negotiate life more successfully. Operating in love is an essential component to the good life!

Day 128

Yes: where two or three come together in my name, I'll be there in the midst of them.—Matthew 18:20

> **Brainy Tip:** Research shows that the love we receive from interacting with others has the power to heal. Yet the converse also applies: people can die from loneliness.

There is just something so powerful about Matthew 18:20. We all know that God never leaves or forsakes us, but it is incredible to think that when we are in a community of love, treating each other with respect, kindness, and compassion, it is as if the Messiah is standing there right next to us. His grace and healing power saturate the room; the presence of true love between people can be incredible. Indeed, our brains and bodies thrive in such an environment, which heals our pains and makes us feel human again. Authentic, unconditional love really does have the power to make all things new!

Day 129

Give, and it will be given to you: a good helping, squashed down, shaken in, and overflowing—that's what will land in your lap. —Luke 6:38

> **Brainy Tip:** Serving others can help you get through tough times, increase your resilience to toxic stress, improve your health, and even increase your longevity.

Many of us, when we are going through hard times, tend to isolate ourselves and say we need "me time." Although it is, of course, healthy to have time alone with your thoughts, escapism is never the answer. Research has shown that caring for others in our state of need actually increases our resilience and reduces our risk of dying! One of the best things we can do when we are going through tough times is to reach out to others in love and serve our community.

There is always someone who needs our help!

Day 130

Then they said, "Come, let us build ourselves a city, and a tower with its top in the heavens, and let us make a name for ourselves."—Genesis 11:4

Brainy Tip: The power of community can be used for good or for ill.

When people come together in the name of love, they can change the world. Yet, as history has shown us, communities also have a dark side. Human beings can form groups and attack people they deem the "other," or they can come together and build an empire that brings hell, not heaven, to earth—think of Nazi Germany, for example. It is incredibly important that we recognize the power of community and how it can be used for good or for evil, to exclude or to love. It is important that we constantly make sure our thoughts, words, and actions measure up to the example of love and inclusiveness we see in the Messiah.

Day 131

Then they said, "Come, let us build ourselves a city, and a tower with its top in the heavens, and let us make a name for ourselves."—Genesis 11:4

Brainy Tip: You create matter with your mind.

Your thinking, feeling, and choosing create matter. Your physical memories are made of proteins that are expressed by your genes, which are switched on or off by your thinking. These thoughts produce fruit: the words and actions that are exclusive to you, which are a construct of your mind.

The question is, what kind of matter are you creating? Are you creating the tower of Babel with your thoughts, worshiping and loving creation rather than the Creator? Or are you creating a city of God, a place where the love of heaven and the beauty of earth meet? Do you live to make a name for yourself or live a life of love? Your mind is incredibly powerful, so be careful how you use it.

Day 132

The Messiah set us free so that we could enjoy freedom! So stand firm, and don't get yourselves tied down by the chains of slavery.—Galatians 5:1

> **Brainy Tip:** We are designed to choose and create—this is the nature of love and the nature of reality, which is shown in the laws of quantum physics.

God has created a probabilistic, open-ended universe. There is an infinite set of possibilities of perception. Although this may sound complicated, it is essentially another way of describing free will and the power of choice. We can choose life or death, blessings or curses.

Quantum physics is a mathematically based description of the open-mindedness of our ability to choose. God uses science to reveal his majesty and the gift of freedom he has given us! And it is up to us whether we let this freedom bring us down or lift us up. We are free to *choose*, so we should do our best to choose wisely to turn positive probabilities into positive realities and avoid the "chains of slavery."

Day 133

Don't let your hearts be troubled; don't be fear-ful.—John 14:27

Brainy Tip: Fear is toxic to the brain and body.

When we are in a constant fear mode, allowing negative probabilities to overtake our minds, we will get caught in a toxic cycle of chemical and neurological responses that influence the choices we make and the reactions we set in motion. Unless we consciously choose to veto and override these reactions, we will voluntarily be at the mercy of the environment, the reactions of our bodies, and the toxic memories of the past.

If we let our fears control us, we will create chaos and disorder in the mind, with all the negative consequences that go with them. However, we do not have to continue down this dark path. We can change, if we choose to use *our minds* to change our brains. We can take back the wheel and redesign our thoughts in alignment with our wired-for-love nature.

Day 134

Be strong and courageous; do not be frightened or dismayed, for the LORD your God is with you wherever you go.
—Joshua 1:9

Brainy Tip: Choosing love over fear can heal your brain and body and help you deal with life. Your genome is designed to respond to your thoughts and words.

Feeling overcome with stress is *not* normal. When we are exposed to or think about something toxic, and there are thought clusters involved with attached toxic emotions, they will set in motion a chemical cascade, launching our minds and bodies into toxic stress mode and affecting our genome.

It is therefore imperative that we learn to control our thinking, taking our thoughts captive and renewing the mind, and in doing so renew our emotions. Don't suppress toxic thoughts or emotions, because they will explode at some point in your life. Choose to have faith in God's strength when you feel like you have no strength left. Rely on his love to help you, and this reliance will enable you to persevere through difficult circumstances.

Day 135

Anxiety weighs down the human heart.—Proverbs 12:25

> **Brainy Tip:** The more you worry and fear something, the more likely that something will come to be.

Every thought changes the brain chemistry, which impacts all 75 to 100 trillion cells of the body at quantum speeds. The impact is instantaneous, literally beyond space and time. An experience of toxic stress and fear can rapidly progress into mental ill health if it is constantly ruminated on and not dealt with. Remember, whatever we think about the most will grow!

Of course, every thought has emotions attached to it; it is important you don't feel bad about feeling! You need to find safe and controlled ways to express these emotions, letting them out by "freaking out in the love zone" and then reconceptualizing them through directed mind action.

Day 136

Throw all your care upon him, because he cares about you.—1 Peter 5:7

Brainy Tip: Mental ill health starts with our thinking.

Mental ill health is not a disease. It is trauma or habituated incorrect thought reactions that have not been dealt with. These thinking patterns create neurological chaos that can manifest as disorders of the mind. Mental ill health starts with the way we react to and deal with life, and can dramatically affect the way we live our lives. It affects everyone because we all have periods in our life when we go through stuff.

It is so important to learn how to control our thinking if we want to develop our mental strength and resilience. When we train ourselves to take our thoughts captive and cast our cares onto God, we can face whatever life throws at us. It will be hard and it will take time, at least sixty-three to eighty-four consecutive days of practice per toxic issue, but it is possible.

Day 137

So don't worry about tomorrow. Tomorrow can worry about itself. One day's trouble at a time is quite enough.
—Matthew 6:34

Brainy Tip: Worrying can cause damage in the brain and body.

Remember, thoughts are *real* things made of proteins that occupy mental real estate. If we worry every day about what might happen or what has happened, we repeatedly re-create the signal that stimulates genetic expression to build and strengthen that thought into a long-term memory. The memory leads to a feeling of uneasiness that produces a toxic stress response that in turn affects our mental and physical health and our relationships.

Train your mind not to ruminate on probabilities that are only possibilities and project them into the future. Possibilities, "what ifs," don't exist until you give them the power to exist through your mind! Do not let worry progress into anxiety and then trauma, because the stronger these fears get, the more time and effort goes into changing them. Nip negative emotions in the bud; don't let them grow like weeds inside your brain.

Day 138

Don't worry about anything. Rather, in every area of life let God know what you want, as you pray and make requests, and give thanks as well.—Philippians 4:6

Brainy Tip: Uncontrolled, negative thinking patterns are toxic to the brain and body.

The more energy we give a toxic thought, the more it grows, and the more we feel consumed and trapped by it. This creates a toxic stress response and will affect us right down to the level of our genes. It will produce toxic fruit in our lives, preventing us from living up to our full potential or bringing heaven to earth through the unique way we think, feel, and choose. We essentially become like broken mirrors, reflecting our pain and fear into the world rather than God's love and grace.

However, the more we focus on God's love, the more we immerse ourselves in his "loveness," the more we can deal with our pain and our fears. The more we speak to the Holy Spirit about what we are going through, and thank him for helping us use the power God has created us with to change and grow, the more we can change the way we think about our past. This new thinking allows us to live up to our full potential in the future.

Day 139

You must bear with one another and, if anyone has a complaint against someone else, you must forgive each other.
—Colossians 3:13

Brainy Tip: Bitterness and unforgiveness can damage the brain.

I do not know what you have been through. I do not know the pain others have caused you, just as you do not know what I have experienced in my life. But I do know, based on both my personal and my professional experience, that it is important to acknowledge how other people have hurt you *and* to forgive these people. If we hold on to our pain, it can develop into a bitter, toxic mindset that can negatively affect the way we think, speak, and function.

Day 140

All bitterness and rage, all anger and yelling, and all blasphemy—put it all away from you, with all wickedness. Instead, be kind to one another, cherish tender feelings for each other, forgive one another, just as God forgave you in the king [Jesus].—Ephesians 4:31–32

Brainy Tip: Forgiveness positively impacts our mental and physical health.

Adopting a forgiveness mindset is a *choice*, an act of your free will. It comes with extreme health benefits. Forgiveness enables you to release toxic thoughts of anger, resentment, bitterness, shame, grief, regret, guilt, and hate. It disentangles you from the source of the issue, removing the negative energy from toxic thinking. People who develop an ability to forgive have greater control over their emotions and are significantly less angry, upset, and hurt and are much healthier!

Day 141

And forgive us the things we owe, as we too have forgiven what was owed to us.—Matthew 6:10

Brainy Tip: When you forgive, you change the structure of your brain in a positive direction.

Forgiveness does not make excuses for someone's behavior. By its nature, forgiveness acknowledges wrongdoing *and*, at the same time, chooses to show grace and mercy. Indeed, forgiveness doesn't mean forgetting, condoning, or excusing whatever happened. Forgiveness acknowledges the pain and reconceptualizes it, releasing the heavy burden of bitterness and resentment.

Day 142

Don't judge, and you won't be judged. Don't condemn, and you won't be condemned. Forgive, and you'll be forgiven.
—Luke 6:37

Brainy Tip: Forgiveness is important for your health.

As a human being who has experienced many painful situations, I know that grace and mercy do not always come easily. Yet it is not important how you forgive, just as long as you do—for your own sake as well as the sake of the people around you. Talking to a friend, therapist, or adviser (spiritual or otherwise) may be helpful during the process, allowing you to sort through your feelings.

Remember, we merge with our environments. Unforgiveness creates a toxic environment. The more you merge with this environment, the more you run the risk of becoming like the issue you are hanging on to.

Day 143

[There is] a time to weep, and a time to laugh; a time to mourn, and a time to dance.—Ecclesiastes 3:4

Brainy Tip: Suppressing emotions can affect your health.

When you express your emotions in a healthy way, including allowing yourself to feel pain when someone hurts you and forgiving your enemies, you allow the free flow of neuropeptides and energy, which in turn allows all bodily systems to function as a healthy whole. However, when you repress and deny your emotions, whatever they may be, you block the network of quantum and chemical pathways, stopping the flow of good chemicals that run your biology and behavior. You will be working against your customized, wired-for-love mode. When you do this for years, you are essentially becoming expert at not feeling what you feel, which can dramatically affect your mental and physical wellbeing.

In life, there are times when you will have to weep, but there are also times when you will laugh and dance. Part of living the good life is recognizing these emotions and expressing them in a healthy way.

Day 144

One who is slow to anger is better than the mighty, and one whose temper is controlled than one who captures a city.—Proverbs 16:32

> **Brainy Tip:** You cannot hide your emotions, but you can learn to control them.

Have you ever thrown a whole lot of clutter into a closet just before guests arrived, only to hear a loud noise as the closet door suddenly opened and everything fell out—in full view of your guests? The same thing can happen in your emotional life. If you repress and hide toxic emotions, the time will come when those buried emotions will suddenly come pouring out. And, of course, it will happen at the most inopportune time, because buried emotions are not controlled, thoughtful emotions. They are volcanic in nature and cannot be suppressed indefinitely. They will explode in some way at some time. Sooner or later, your emotions will come out, so you have to learn how to express your emotions in a healthy and controlled way by controlling the way you think about what you are facing.

Day 145

Like a city breached, without walls, is one who lacks self-control.—Proverbs 25:28

Brainy Tip: Uncontrolled emotions are toxic to the brain and body.

Each thought has its own chemical signature—your thinking quite literally becomes a feeling with a resultant chemical reaction in your brain and body. When you step out of your wired-for-love design, your thoughts and emotions become unbalanced and toxic. If these toxic feelings dominate, a neurochemical rush can start to distort them in the direction of fear, which can result in toxic stress and cause damage in the brain and body.

Indeed, out-of-control emotions will completely block your ability to think things through with wisdom and insight. Submitting to them causes chemical chaos in the brain and makes your mind foggy. You will lose concentration and find it difficult to listen to anything anyone is trying to say to you. You can spiral into a black hole quickly if you do not use your powerful mind to deliberately and intentionally capture these thoughts and reconceptualize them.

Day 146

Jesus burst into tears.—John 11:35

Brainy Tip: We are made to feel and express a wide range of emotions.

Many of us have become experts at hiding our emotions. Signs of suppressed feelings include conflict, irritability, short temper, over-reactivity, anxiety, frustration, fear, impulsiveness, a desire for control, perfectionism, and self-doubt. Acknowledging that we are expressing emotions is an important step in detoxing our mind and brain. If we continue to try to hide what we feel, we will block our path to success in life.

Even Jesus experienced grief at times! Indeed, many mental health problems stem from an inability to express our emotions, incorrectly dealing with our feelings, or numbing them with psychotropic drugs. The thoughts with their attached emotions won't just go away with medication or suppression. They have to be brought into the conscious mind from the nonconscious mind and reconceptualized (changed); the incorrect thinking habit has to be eliminated mentally and physically.

The more we learn to trust and praise God in the midst of our problems and during the happy times, just as Jesus did, the more we will be better equipped, mentally and physically, to deal with the vagaries of life.

Day 147

I am about to do a new thing; now it springs forth, do you not perceive it? I will make a way in the wilderness and rivers in the desert.—Isaiah 43:19

> **Brainy Tip:** We can change our past by allowing the future to reach back. This is called retroactive causation in quantum physics. It essentially shows us how "loveness" and prayer are beyond space and time.

There is always hope. Regardless of the way you have chosen to react in the past, painful toxic thoughts can be reconstructed. You can reconstruct even toxic feelings you have been nursing for so long and are so familiar that you think they are normal. You can analyze them and rewire them because of the brain's neuroplasticity. You *can* change the way you think about and react to the circumstances of life. With the help of the Holy Spirit, you can "make a way in the wilderness and rivers in the desert."

When we pray, we pray not only for the future but also to change the past and to retell our story through the eyes of Jesus's love. We can actually change our past by allowing the future of God's hope to reach back into our lives. This is called retroactive causation, and it essentially shows us how "loveness" and prayer are beyond space and time. You never have to be a victim of what you have said or done or what others have said about you or done to you.

Remember, nothing is impossible for God. He has given you a truly phenomenal mind!

Day 148

God has bestowed upon us, through his divine power, everything that we need for life and godliness, through the knowledge of him who called us by his own glory and virtue.—2 Peter 1:3

> **Brainy Tip:** You can control the way you think, feel, and choose—this is evident in both Scripture and science. You need to choose to really believe and apply this to your life.

It may sound daunting to try to capture all of your thoughts and control your emotions. Yet when you understand how you can scientifically choose, in an organized way,[1] what becomes a part of who you are (your Perfect You[2]), you will begin to understand that you have an amazing ability to change and overcome.

We all have the opportunity to choose to walk in the Perfect You God has given us, despite our circumstances. Once you learn how to think in love and listen to the Holy Spirit, allowing him to guide your mind, you can tap into the amazing power for transformation God has given you, and nothing will seem impossible!

Day 149

Focus the mind on the flesh, and you'll die; but focus it on the spirit, and you'll have life, and peace.—Romans 8:6

Brainy Tip: What we choose to think about matters!

Our thoughts have the capacity to affect the actions of our brains and bodies because of the divinely invested power in our design. Our free will is rooted and grounded in feelings of worth and value—we matter, and what we think matters. And what we think, feel, and choose changes matter. We are one hundred percent responsible for what we choose to think about.

Where we choose to direct our attention creates realities in our lives. When we choose to follow the example of love we see in the Messiah, we bring life and peace into the world. When we choose to focus on and worship the pleasures the kingdoms of the world offer, such as sex, food, money, and power, we bring pain, death, and destruction into the world. The choice is ours, so choose life.

Day 150

Whatever you do, do it with love.—1 Corinthians 16:14

> **Brainy Tip:** Love can change the way the brain and body function. Loving others and being loved changes the blood chemistry in all 75 to 100 trillion cells of the brain and body!

When we operate in love, our brains respond in the way they are designed to respond. Loving others and being loved actually changes the blood chemistry in all 75 to 100 trillion cells of our brains and bodies. Based on the information we get from brain technology (which, we need to bear in mind, is limited), we can see that areas of the corpus striatum will be activated more than other areas, neurotransmitters and peptides and hormones will be secreted, and we will feel good and be able to rejoice despite our circumstances.

Love is extremely powerful. When you choose to operate in unconditional love, you change yourself—spirit, mind, and body—as well as those with whom you are in relationship and even the earth.

Day 151

Every person should be quick to hear, slow to speak, slow to anger.—James 1:19

> **Brainy Tip:** We are not preprogrammed biological robots. We control our attitudes.

Every time we think, we release quantum energy and chemicals in response. These produce feelings and reactions in the body. Clusters of electromagnetic and quantum energy embossed in proteins form thoughts with attached chemical messengers, which form the substrate of our memories inside the brain. In turn, these collectively form attitudes.

We express our attitudes—based in love or toxic fear—through our Perfect You via what we think, feel, and choose. We can therefore control our attitudes by controlling our thinking—we are not slaves to our feelings. We are not preprogrammed biological robots. We can't blame our genes, brain, or parents for our attitudes—we need to take responsibility for what we think. We are able to listen, speak, and react *in love*, if we choose to do so.

Day 152

Anyone who doesn't love abides in death.—1 John 3:14

> **Brainy Tip:** Toxic thinking blocks cognitive flexibility and deep intellectual thought.

If you have a toxic thought while you are processing information in your own unique way, you have to push that information through the toxic thoughts (toxic attitude) in your brain. Toxic thoughts and their tangible bad attitude block your Perfect You—who you are at your core. In turn, operating outside of the Perfect You, which essentially means operating outside of your wired-for-love design, inhibits your ability to think and operate in wisdom, thereby inhibiting your overall health, mentally and physically. When we do not love, we bring "death" and decay into our lives.

Day 153

No creature remains hidden before God. All are naked, laid bare before the eyes of the one to whom we must present an account.—Hebrews 4:13

Brainy Tip: You cannot hide what consumes your mind.

Attitudes reflect the core of how you are spending your time thinking, feeling, and choosing. They reflect your spiritual development and what you are doing with your power, love, and sound mind in a causal way. They reflect what you think about the most—what you *worship*.

What we choose to think about the most, where we choose to let our mind wander, and what we love and worship cannot be hidden. God sees what is in our hearts (minds), and what is in our minds will affect what we think, say, and do—the fruit of our life.

What kind of account will you give to God when it comes to your thinking?

Day 154

Love is the greatest.—1 Corinthians 13:13

Brainy Tip: We are wired for love, and we have to learn toxic fear, because this kind of negative fear is not our default mode; love is our default mode.

Fear may be powerful if we give it energy through our thinking, feeling, and choosing, but it is important to remember that love is much more powerful and our brains were made to operate in love. Perfect love can overcome fear, because God is love. Love is the foundation of all existence, and so the absence of love is merely a type of nonexistence—it is a destructive, chaotic void that has no power over our lives unless we give it power over our lives.

Day 155

Turn away from evil and do good . . . seek peace, and follow after it.—1 Peter 3:11

> **Brainy Tip:** We can choose to be at peace, regardless of our circumstances.

Each of us has our own electrical chemical balance where we are at peace. We need to constantly seek after this peace by remembering that we cannot control our circumstances (life and people) but *we can choose to control our reactions* (attitudes) to those circumstances.

The more we seek out and follow this peace, allowing it to guide our thinking, the more we will turn away from "evil" reactions such as bitterness, hatred, and unforgiveness, and the more we will manifest God's goodness in our lives through our wise decisions and reactions.

Day 156

This, you see, is how much God loved the world: enough to give his only, special son, so that everyone who believes in him should not be lost but should share in the life of God's new age.—John 3:16

Brainy Tip: We see from the study of quantum physics that love is the basic reality of consciousness and that love necessitates the freedom of choice.

If you focus on only your fears or concerns, you will block your Perfect You—you will never truly feel like you. Your brain and body will respond to your choices and distort the love circuit into the fear circuit.

However, even though fear is powerful, operating in love is even more powerful. Love, after all, has the power to restore and renew the world. And you can choose. You are not a victim of your circumstances or your biology. You have the choice to operate in God's love or in worry, fear, and anxiety within your circumstances.

Day 157

This is how you should think among yourselves—with the mind that you have because you belong to the Messiah, Jesus.—Philippians 2:5

> **Brainy Tip:** Love incorporates a specific way of thinking that each of us has at the core of who we are, a type of thinking that is part of a bigger picture: the reflection of God's love through humanity on earth.

When we begin to recognize how powerful our unique choices are, how powerful the "mind [we] have because [we] belong to the Messiah" is, we can begin to tap into this power, not only for us but also for the world around us.

When we follow the example of love we see in Jesus, we truly begin to understand the *responsibility* we have to act in our divine, wired-for-love state. We each have a role to play that no one else can play, and if we don't operate in our particular "love zone," the whole world is impacted. Each of us is a piece in the puzzle that is life!

It is no wonder that the apostle Paul constantly tells us to follow the example of love we see in the Messiah. It's also time for us to start realizing our role in humanity and step up to the plate. It's not about "me, myself, and I." It's about *me in the world.*

Think of Paul's life. How did he think, act, and speak in love? How did he use his incredible mind to change the world? What does love look like in your life? How can you step into your wired-for-love design?

Day 158

And you have put on the new one—which is being renewed in the image of the creator, bringing you into possession of new knowledge.—Colossians 3:10

Brainy Tip: Humans play a pivotal role in quantum physics, because it is human choice that leads to change.

Our minds are creative forces to be reckoned with and are to be used in the best ways possible. We have to constantly watch our thoughts, put on our new selves, and make sure we use our image-bearing "loveness" in positive ways. We need to ask the Holy Spirit for wisdom, "new knowledge," that will enable us to renew our minds and change the way we live.

We need to reflect the image of a loving God, not a broken world order. What we choose to do with our minds—our thinking, feeling, and choosing—will bring heaven or hell to earth.

The question is, whose image are you reflecting?

Day 159

We must all appear before the judgment seat of God.—Romans 14:10

Brainy Tip: Choice is an important responsibility.

As image-bearers of God, with a responsibility to steward creation, we are so much more than the firing of our neurons. And creation incorporates all of humanity, with our spirits, minds, and bodies, and this incredible earth, with all its vegetation and animals. We have been tasked with caring for *all* of creation so that God may be glorified.

What we choose is reflected in the activity of our brains—our brains are responding to our minds. What we choose cannot be reduced to the activity of our brains. As Oxford professor and philosopher Richard Swinburne notes, "our mental lives cannot be captured in purely physical terms."[1] Neuroscience can further bits of information, such as the mechanism by which a lack of food kindles the desire to eat, yet neuroscience has never shown, nor will show, the choice of a person to act on his or her desires, or to choose whether to do good or evil.

The Bible, from Adam and Eve in Genesis to the book of Revelation, constantly emphasizes the fact that our choices are powerful and can lead to life or death. Being human means accepting this responsibility to take our thoughts captive and constantly reflect the image of a loving God into creation, because we *will be held accountable* for the impact of our choices.

We love the freedom of choice, but do we love its consequences?

Day 160

"You must love the Lord your God," replied Jesus, "with all your heart, with all your life, and with all your mind."
—Matthew 22:37

Brainy Tip: Your mind will only change your brain in the right direction when you operate in God's "loveness."

Each of us think, feel, and choose with our minds. Neuroscience and classical physics only describe the physical response of the brain to the mind-in-action, the mind being the first cause. The brain is the substrate through which the mind works—it reflects the action of the mind. The mind controls the brain; the brain does not control the mind. We are not victims of our biology. Through our thoughts, we can change our biology.

When we learn to love God with our whole person, including our mind, we use the power we have in our minds for good. We can create realities that bring heaven to earth as we reflect his image into the world.

Day 161

But you are "a chosen race; a royal priesthood"; a holy nation; a people for God's possession. Your purpose is to announce the virtuous deeds of the one who called you out of darkness into his amazing light.—1 Peter 2:9

Brainy Tip: Science confirms that there is no one like you with your unique perceptions, unique God-given energy, and unique expression of consciousness.

You are special. Although this may sound like a silly, overused cliché, it is nevertheless true. You are unique. You have a particular way of thinking, feeling, and choosing that acts like a filter through which you experience reality; this is your individual stream of consciousness. It shapes the worldview you build into your mind, which in turn shapes your future thoughts, feelings, words, and behavior. You reflect a unique part of the image of God. If you are not you, the world does not get to experience a special part of God's loving divinity.

You are a member of a "chosen race, a royal priesthood." You "announce the virtuous deeds of the one who called you out of darkness into his amazing light" by doing just that: choosing to embrace and reflect the unique light he has placed inside of you by being the person he called you to be.

Day 162

Every one of you should test your own work, and then you will have a reason to boast of yourself, not of somebody else. Each of you, you see, will have to carry your own load.
—Galatians 6:4–5

Brainy Tip: Envying and imitating others will cause brain damage and negatively impact your health.

You make a wonderful you but a lousy someone else. Envying other people and trying to make a different filter fit the way you are designed—that is, trying to be, act, or live like someone else—will distort your worldview and ability to think, feel, and choose, which will impact your mental and physical health and prevent you from living up to your full potential.

Indeed, when you are not you, the world suffers. You have a special work to do; you have something unique and wonderful to give to the world. "Test your own work," and be proud of your own perfect youness. Don't sell yourself short. Don't let the world miss out on what you have to give.

Day 163

That's how it is with the son of man: he didn't come to have servants obey him, but to be a servant—and to give his life as "a ransom for many."—Matthew 20:28

Brainy Tip: We are designed to serve others. Serving others will change how our bodies and brains function right down to the level of our DNA and quantum energy.

If you want to live the good life, you have to learn to follow the servant model of the Messiah. This not just something nice to say or to teach in leadership training; this is essential to a life well lived, the most meaningful life you can live.

There truly is no point in being talented or unique (that is, your Perfect You) if you live in a one-person universe, which is actually toxic to your brain and body. Your Perfect You locks down in isolation but flourishes as a part of God's body. Your entanglement in the lives of others enhances the quality of your own life.

In the current world (including the church!) a "me, myself, and I" mindset of self-motivation and selfishness is too often the focus of our desires, prayers, and worship. We often treat God like a slot machine, complaining when he doesn't give us what we want because we put the coins of good behavior or nice words in. But life is not about what God must do for you; it's about what *you* can do for others. When you think with a servant mindset, your love nature is activated, and happiness and peace can flow into your life.

Day 164

Teach me good judgment and knowledge.—Psalm 119:66

> **Brainy Tip:** Quantum physics shows that we are to receive wisdom from a supreme source.

A memory is built when genetic expression happens, which occurs as we *choose*. Choosing makes physical thoughts come into being—you create matter with your mind.

Your brain is designed to respond to knowledge, and you need to detect whether this information is good or bad for you; otherwise you will build toxic knowledge into your brain with your mind. This toxic knowledge can influence your thoughts, words, and actions in the future. This is why it is so important to set up a constant communication with the Spirit in order to access the wisdom of God, the supreme source of all existence, whose judgment and knowledge are always good.

Day 165

Return to the LORD, your God, for he is gracious and merciful, slow to anger, and abounding in steadfast love, and relents from punishing.—Joel 2:13

Brainy Tip: It is never too late to change your thinking.

Do you feel like you are stuck in a rut? Do you want to change but feel like change is impossible? You are not a victim of your thoughts or your biology; you are a victor over them. This means you can change your thoughts! You may have been nursing negative mindsets for so long that they are familiar to you and you think they are normal. This mistake is often made. However, only the thoughts formed when you are in your Perfect You, from God's perspective, are normal, while the rest need redesigning or, to use the scientific term, reconceptualization. You can analyze your thoughts and, because of the neuroplasticity of the brain, redesign and rewire them. You can embrace your wired-for-love design! It is never too late to change your thinking.

Day 166

Let us then come boldly to the throne of grace, so that we may receive mercy, and may find grace to help us at the moment when we need it.—Hebrews 4:16

Brainy Tip: You can observe and change the way you think. This ability to stand outside yourself and observe yourself is called the multiple perspective advantage, which generates activity in the front of the brain.

You *can* analyze your thoughts and self-regulate what you are thinking, feeling, and choosing—and what to say and do—because of the neuroplasticity of the brain. You are also able to redesign and rewire your thoughts and therefore change your words and actions. This is grace meeting science!

Indeed, research shows that conscious awareness of thoughts makes them amenable to change because they are physically weakened. This is called the multiple perspective advantage (MPA). When toxic thoughts are weak, they can be reconceptualized, bringing life back into the brain and body. When you bring these toxic thoughts into conscious awareness, analyze them, and change them, you harness the power that is in your mind!

Day 167

I'm telling you the truth: if you have faith like a grain of mustard seed, you will say to this mountain, "Move from here to there," and it will move. Nothing will be impossible for you.—Matthew 17:20

Brainy Tip: When you gain insight into your consciousness, which can change mind into matter and effect behavioral changes, you will gain insight into "mustard seed" faith. It is possible to change the way you think and change the way you live your life.

It may, of course, sound daunting to try to capture all of your attitudes and constantly observe your thinking, but both science and Scripture show that this is the design of your mind and brain. As you develop your understanding of how you can scientifically choose what becomes a part of who you are, you will also understand that you have an amazing opportunity to be the person the Creator designed you to be. "You will say to this mountain, 'Move from here to there,' and it will move." *It will move!*

After all, nothing is impossible for God. So do not try to make God fit into the small box of your imagination, because there isn't even a box to begin with!

Day 168

One who is cool in spirit has understanding.—Proverbs 17:27

Brainy Tip: You need to be aware of what is going on in your head to change the way you think.

Mindful awareness of what is going on in your mind—that is, a willing and intentional awareness to turn toward your inner spirit, mind, and body experiences—is a far more effective way to handle toxic stress than trying to change your toxic reactions in a mindless, ad hoc, and reactive way. Thinking about your thinking allows you to remain calm and collected in the midst of difficult circumstances and apply the wisdom that you will gain to tough problems.

Day 169

People whose lives are determined by human flesh focus their minds on matters to do with the flesh, but people whose lives are determined by the spirit focus their minds on matters to do with the spirit. Focus the mind on the flesh, and you'll die; but focus it on the spirit, and you'll have life, and peace.—Romans 8:5–6

Brainy Tip: We are spiritual beings with minds that exist in the spiritual world as well as material beings with bodies and brains that exist in a material world. We have a strong sense of intuition because of this connection, and we can develop it through mental practice.

Every time we face a decision, we are in an "about to choose" state (known as superposition in quantum physics). If we choose to ask the Holy Spirit to help us focus in this state, we can calm down, let go, and step back as we become aware of the need for his wisdom and guidance. We increase our intuitive powers, almost standing outside ourselves, and the crazy chaos of our thinking calms down. In this state, we can make wise and loving choices, which bring life and peace into the world. We can connect the spiritual and physical realms of existence, bringing a piece of heaven to earth.

Day 170

What will happen, though, is that you will receive power when the holy spirit comes upon you. Then you will be my witnesses in Jerusalem, in all Judaea and Samaria, and to the very ends of the earth.—Acts 1:8

Brainy Tip: God has given us everything we need to choose well.

When we make a choice, our emotional perceptual library (the amygdala) does not always provide the accurate truth, because it works on perceptions we have built into our minds through our choices and reactions, and human perceptions are sometimes false. In fact, the emotions stored in this library can be quite dangerous if we allow them to control us.

So what should we do to choose well? We need to mindfully and intentionally remind ourselves that God has given us everything we need. He has given us a way to handle every situation, so we should not make choices without him. In superposition (the quantum term for the type of limbo state that exists before a decision is made), we need to consciously ask God for wisdom and focus on the fruits of the Spirit so we can truly be witnesses of his amazing love and power as we think, feel, and choose. We need to get in a rhythm with the Spirit!

Day 171

But the helper, the holy spirit, the one the father will send in my name, he will teach you everything. He will bring back to your mind everything I've said to you.—John 14:26

> **Brainy Tip:** We are designed to think about our thinking.

When we ask the Holy Spirit for wisdom in superposition, we take advantage of a circuit God has built into our brains that runs between the amygdala and the front part of the brain called the prefrontal cortex (PFC), which is situated more or less behind the eyebrows. Operating much like a scale, this circuit responds to balance reason and emotion. This is because the frontal lobe, of which the PFC is a part, is directly connected to all the other parts of the brain and therefore becomes very active when we mindfully self-regulate. The PFC also has at its command the basal forebrain, which activates all the processing loops through the brain. It manages, coordinates, and integrates all other brain regions when the mind is in action through thinking, feeling, and choosing.

The PFC is very active when we reason and understand our own thoughts about ourselves. We do this by reasoning out the situation facing us, in our minds or out loud, almost as though we were standing outside ourselves thinking about our thinking and asking the Holy Spirit to guide our thinking. This is taking thoughts captive in action!

Day 172

People who remain in me, and I in them, are the ones who bear plenty of fruit. Without me, you see, you can't do anything.—John 15:5

> **Brainy Tip:** Our thoughts can affect the entire body almost instantaneously through quantum energy and the flow of chemicals.

Acknowledging our thoughts, feelings, existing memories, and bodily reactions is of paramount importance, because the emotions are dynamic chemicals that flow in the bloodstream between cells and deposit information about the memory into cells. This also happens through quantum action, because the brain is like a biological quantum computer.

If you suppress an emotion, it will explode somewhere. The hypothalamic-pituitary-adrenal (HPA) axis will be disrupted and function abnormally. This HPA16 axis involves the hypothalamus and pituitary glands in the brain and the adrenal glands just above the kidneys. It is the circuit that is activated in a complex, cyclic way of tension and release as we are responding to life all day long. Our thoughts can affect the entire body in an instant!

As frightening and overwhelming as this may sound, we need to remember that we are designed to ask the Holy Spirit for help. We don't have to deal with life alone! With the help of the Messiah, we can deal with anything that comes our way. If we try to sort out all our issues alone, we can end up in an even bigger mess. Without him, we cannot do anything well.

Day 173

Don't you know that when people run on the racetrack everybody runs, but only one person gets the prize? Run in such a way that you'll win it.—1 Corinthians 9:24

> **Brainy Tip:** We have a natural pharmacopeia inside of us, as well as a quantum and genetic design that is powerful enough to help us overcome whatever comes our way.

Once we realize that we control our pain, toxic thinking, and wrong feelings and reactions, and once we truly understand that these do not control us, we are set free to start running God's race and reflecting his glorious image.

We all have the opportunity to choose to walk in the Perfect You God has given us, despite our circumstances. We don't have to get stuck in the pain and tragedy of the past or the present. We can move forward by "freaking out in the love zone!"

Day 174

Let your hand be ready to help me, for I have chosen your precepts.—Psalm 119:173

> **Brainy Tip:** Quantum physics, with its examination of science beyond the traditional paradigms of space and time, points directly to the belief that the universe has a creative mind behind it (consciousness), and therefore a creative purpose.

When you choose to follow the way of love, the creative mind of God, you are going to realize what it means to always be in a "genesis moment." Every time you think, it actively changes your brain and body either for better (within your Perfect You) or worse (outside your Perfect You).

When you make bad choices, toxic thought clusters with their attached emotions cause you to step out of your Perfect You, and this slippage affects your thoughts, words, and actions. However, every time you operate according to your Perfect You, you are operating in your perfect design, reflecting a particular part of God's image. If you choose to follow the example of love we see in the Messiah, you choose to allow God to help you and give you wisdom. You essentially choose to activate the genesis power within you in a positive, life-giving way.

What do you want activated in your life today, tomorrow, and for the rest of your life? What do you want to create?

Day 175

No discipline seems to bring joy at the time, but only sorrow. Later, though, it produces fruit, the peaceful fruit of righteousness, for those who are trained by it.—Hebrews 12:11

Brainy Tip: The more you practice taking your thoughts captive, the more you will take your thoughts captive. This requires daily disciplined, intentional, and deliberate practice in cycles of twenty-one days.[1]

Practice being aware of what you are thinking. Practice bringing all thoughts into captivity. Don't let any thoughts go unchecked through your mind. Stop randomly thinking and be intentional in what you choose to think about. Do this every day in cycles of twenty-one days.

Take the time to sort out your thinking before your thinking gets the best of you! It may be a difficult process, and it may cause you sorrow, but in the end you will experience the joy of being free from the negative strongholds in your life. You will experience the joy of being who you were created to be!

Day 176

After he had sent the crowds away, Jesus went up the mountain by himself to pray.—Matthew 14:23

Brainy Tip: Alone time helps you observe your own thinking.

I cannot stress how important it is for your brain to have "thinker time." Find some periods of alone time, just for thinking—no phone, iPad, computer, people, or other distractions—just you sitting still, thinking. Do this for at least one to two minutes each day. It may be a bit of a challenge at first, but stick with it!

As you quietly think deeply, you are gaining insight into the way you think, which is fundamental to introspection, self-knowledge, and understanding your own feelings, thoughts, and intuitions. Take the time to talk to the Holy Spirit, asking him to guide you as you observe your own thinking. This deep, intellectual thinking improves brain health, reboots the brain, and brings order to the mind.

Day 177

Look at the remarkable love the father has given us—that we should be called God's children! That indeed is what we are.—1 John 3:1

Brainy Tip: Your brain is designed to build meaningful thoughts; otherwise it becomes toxic.

Your life has meaning. When we begin to see who we are, our blueprint for identity, we begin to discover the meaning of our lives.

Meaning is not just something that happens inside our brains. It is something that evolves through the Perfect You and provides context to the things that come into our lives. Our thoughts, feelings, choices, words, experiences, lives— these all have meaning, which is beautifully shaped and expressed through the special way each of us thinks, feels, and chooses.

What an honor to live as a child of God! You really do matter. What you think matters. Do not let anyone tell you otherwise.

Day 178

How much do five sparrows cost? Two copper coins? And not one of them is forgotten in God's presence. But the hairs of your head have all been counted. Don't be afraid! You are worth more than lots of sparrows.—Luke 12:6–7

Brainy Tip: Self-esteem is the key to making a difference in the world because it emphasizes the unique contribution of each human being.

You are a high priest of creation. This means you are a very important person! Low self-esteem underlies the vast majority of mind issues, but it doesn't have to! God loves you. You are designed to glorify his name; you are created to love and to reach beyond yourself. Every thought you think is a veritable universe and has a powerful impact in the world.

But you cannot grow into the fullest expression of yourself if you live in a state of doubt or internal unrest. You need to believe in and love yourself, and trust in the God who created you, if you want to change the world for the better.

Day 179

People don't light a lamp and put it under a bucket; they put it on a lampstand. Then it gives light to everybody in the house. That's how you must shine your light in front of people! Then they will see what wonderful things you do, and they'll give glory to your father in heaven.—Matthew 5:15–16

Brainy Tip: You have something unique and wonderful to give to the world.

The world is all about probabilities. You, with your Perfect You, are at the intersection of making your unique probabilities real and meaningful because no one can see what you see. It is your personal experience. And as you create a unique reality with your brilliant Perfect You, you are updating your knowledge of the world and adding a quality to the world that only you can add.

You are not designed to collide with everyone else's experience. You are designed to walk alongside everyone else in your uniqueness. It is not the world or us but rather us within the world. Your unique mind, expressed through your Perfect You, reflects God's glory, bringing heaven to earth and making the world a more beautiful place. You are a light, so don't hide yourself under a basket!

Day 180

We have the mind of the Messiah.—*1 Corinthians 2:16*

Brainy Tip: We have power to make physically efficacious decisions on the basis of reason and evaluations.

God created the universe and its laws and has given part of his power to human beings, who are created in his own image. Like God, we have power to create realities through our choices. We can create changes in our brains and in our worlds.

Each of us has this extraordinary ability to determine, achieve, and maintain optimal levels of intelligence, mental health, peace, and happiness, as well as the prevention of disease in our bodies and minds. Each of us has the powerful, life-giving, miracle-creating mind of the Messiah. We can, through conscious effort and intellectual reasoning, gain control of our thoughts and feelings, and in doing so, we can change the programming and chemistry of our brains.

This is an incredible yet rewarding challenge. Are you up to it?

Day 181

So take special care how you conduct yourselves. Don't be unwise, but be wise.—Ephesians 5:15

Brainy Tip: Wise thinking results in increased clarity of thought, clearness of vision, intellectual processing, emotional balance, and improved physical health.

Breakthrough neuroscientific research is confirming daily what we have instinctively known all along: what you are thinking every moment of every day becomes a physical reality in your brain and body, which affects your optimal mental and physical health.

Wise thinking produces a mindset that is able to examine all factors and perspectives related to thinking, feeling, and choosing. It is the key to understanding your psyche, your personhood, and the uniqueness of your actions and reactions. It activates your consciousness, which is your divine sense of purpose. It kindles your courage and thus your determination to achieve your dreams.

Day 182

O that you had paid attention to my commandments! Then your prosperity would have been like a river, and your success like the waves of the sea.—Isaiah 48:18

> **Brainy Tip:** When we self-reflect, we activate the physical brain to function at a higher intellectual level.

Your state of mind is a real, physical, electromagnetic, quantum, and chemical flow in the brain that switches groups of genes on or off in a positive or negative direction based on your choices and subsequent reactions. Scientifically, this is called epigenetics; spiritually, this is known as free will. The brain responds to your mind by sending neurological signals throughout your body, which means that your thoughts and emotions are transformed into physiological and spiritual effects, and then physiological experiences transform into mental and emotional states.

Although you may recognize what I am saying from previous days, the science bears repeating. The way the mind works is an incredible gift from an incredible God, and when you begin to understand and realize what a gift this is, you truly begin to understand what "prosperity" looks like in your own life when you follow the love of God. I found in my clinical practice that awareness was the key to my patients taking ownership of their lives. It's a profound and eye-opening thought to realize something as seemingly immaterial as a belief can take on a physical existence as a positive or negative change in our cells.

Day 183

You see, nothing is hidden which won't become visible; nothing is concealed that won't come to light.—Luke 8:17

Brainy Tip: Thinking in action creates structural change in the brain, which in turn makes the unseen visible through your words and actions.

Your brain responds to your mind by sending neurological signals in your body. Your thoughts and emotions are transformed into physiological and spiritual effects. In turn, your physiological experiences are transformed into mental and emotional states—everything is connected when it comes to the mind.

You really cannot blame anyone else for what you say and do. Although people and situations can certainly influence your decisions, ultimately God has put you in charge of your mind, and he advises you to get his help in managing it (the Holy Spirit)!

Day 184

Yet you have made them a little lower than God, and crowned them with glory and honor.—Psalm 8:5

Brainy Tip: Neurologically, the power of "loveness" we have from God activates the reward thinking/learning circuit in the brain.

These readings are designed to help you discover who you are and what you can do. I want you to literally plumb the depths of who you are and get to understand the value God has vested in you as his wonderful creation.

Think of your ability to think and choose and to use your mind. Even though changing your mind by renewing it is often the hardest step in changing the way you live your life, it is also the first and most powerful step. In fact, without this step, nothing else will work and you will keep "going around the mountain."

If, however, you consciously direct your thinking, you can wire out toxic patterns of thinking and replace them with life-giving, healthy thoughts. New thought networks will grow, saturating your brain with the glory of the Creator. You will increase your intelligence and bring healing to your brain, mind, and physical body.

It all starts in the realm of the mind, with your ability to think and choose—the most powerful thing in the universe after God, and, indeed, fashioned after God.

Day 185

The thief only comes to steal, and kill, and destroy. I came so that they could have life—yes, and have it full to overflowing.—John 10:10

> **Brainy Tip:** Lies have no power unless we give them power.

It is with our minds that we reject or believe the lies of the satan. Lies are not realities; lies are *probabilities* of what can be. It is with our minds that we turn these probabilities into physical realities as a thought network made of proteins in our brains, a network that affects what we say and do and how we perceive the world.

When we choose to listen to the lies of the satan, we give them substance and energy. We literally create sin inside our heads because we have turned a nothing (the lie) into a something! This is a sobering reality, because we often ask ourselves where evil comes from. If we believe that Jesus conquered sin and death and evil, then this evil no longer has power. So why is there still human evil? We, as human beings made in the image of God, abuse our ability to choose and create evil realities in our heads instead of love-based realities that reflect the glory of our Creator.

Day 186

Death, where's your victory gone? Death, where's your sting gone?—1 Corinthians 15:55

Brainy Tip: It is never too late to change the way you think.

The brain is neuroplastic. Neuroplasticity by definition means the brain is malleable and adaptable, changing moment by moment of every day. Neuroplasticity shows that God designed our brains to change as we renew our minds—how marvelous and generous! Scientists are finally beginning to see the brain as having renewable characteristics; it is no longer viewed as a machine that is hardwired early in life, unable to adapt, and wearing out with age. With example after fascinating example, exceptional scientists talk about and demonstrate—using brain-imaging techniques and the evidence of behavioral changes—how people can change their brains with their minds.

So, no matter where you are in life, don't give up hope. Don't stop running the race that God has set before you! You can change. You can overcome. You are not your past; you are not your present. You are what you choose to be—what you choose to focus on the most. Death and fear do not have power over you, unless you give them that power.

Day 187

The LORD, the LORD, a God merciful and gracious, slow to anger, and abounding in steadfast love and faithfulness, keeping steadfast love for the thousandth generation, forgiving iniquity and transgression and sin, yet by no means clearing the guilty, but visiting the iniquity of the parents upon the children and the children's children, to the third and the fourth generation.—Exodus 34:6–7

> **Brainy Tip:** What you think affects your descendants—this is called epigenetics.

How we think not only affects our own spirit, soul, and body but also people around us. Science (epigenetics) and Scripture both show how the results of our decisions pass through the sperm and ova to the next four generations at least, profoundly affecting their choices and lifestyles.

What kind of "thinking" inheritance will you leave your children and your children's children?

Day 188

Human eyes are never satisfied.—Proverbs 27:20

Brainy Tip: You are as content as you want to be.

The fact that the brain can change (neuroplasticity) and rebuild new nerve cells (neurogenesis) is both exciting and incredibly hopeful! It means happiness comes from within and success follows—not the other way around.

Indeed, you don't have to have the latest iPhone, or Mercedes sedan, or a 62-inch television to be happy. You are not a slave to how many likes you get on Instagram. You are not happy only if you have a six-figure income. You are as happy and content as you want to be, right now, right where you are in life. Relying on possessions that eventually lose their value or the fleeting approval of people will leave you in a dark place—such desires will never satisfy.

Day 189

An intelligent mind acquires knowledge, and the ear of the wise seeks knowledge.—Proverbs 18:15

Brainy Tip: You are as intelligent as you want to be.

Your brain operates like a biological quantum computer. Every day you need to detox your thought life and strengthen and build your brain through deep thinking and intellectual pursuits.

How do you do this? Watch your thinking, renew your mind, and *learn something new every day*. I spend up to two hours each day learning new information in my field, not only because I love this information but also because it is very good for my brain and body.[1] You can learn how to learn and deepen your intellect. You can overcome any learning issues you have been told you have. You can get the chaos in your mind under control. You can *learn* to think well!

Day 190

Along with the testing, he will provide the way of escape, so that you can bear it.—1 Corinthians 10:13

Brainy Tip: How you *understand and use* your mind is predictive of how successful you will be.

We define our own success. These readings are all about helping you get to that place that allows you to succeed in all areas of your life—to find that "switch" for a life well lived, a life that is filled with *meaningful* success that reflects the glory of God into the world. This book is about mental self-care. It takes you beyond mindfulness into a lifestyle of cognitive transformation that is both sustainable and organic—suited to your Perfect You.

Mental self-care is integrally interwoven into a life of meaning, which naturally evolves into success in school, work, and every other area of your life. It is the key to finding your vocation or purpose: what gets you out of bed in the morning and every morning to come. It is therefore the key to recognizing that God has given you what you need. You just need to learn how to access what God has given you!

Day 191

In all toil there is profit, but mere talk leads only to poverty.—Proverbs 14:23

Brainy Tip: Changing the brain is hard but rewarding work. It is essential for mental self-care.

We need to make our brains work for us and not against us. We need to get our minds working properly again. Mental self-care incorporates understanding and using the power of the mind to build useful memory *with understanding*. This is not rote learning or memory tricks or Twitter thinking. Healthy, productive learning is good, old-fashioned hard work that draws on the amazing capacity we have as humans to think and learn.

To succeed, we need to take responsibility for thinking and learning. No one is going to do it for us. We shouldn't be tempted to fall for the gadgets, gizmos, tricks, or DIY guides that promise to make us smarter and more intelligent *overnight*. Nothing will ever replace diligent, intentional, conscious, and corrective hard work. Only mind activity will change the brain, which will produce changes in what we say and do. This change requires discipline. The dangers of the current environment we live in have made us impatient, a trifle entitled, and mostly unwilling to sacrifice and work hard.

Time and effort are the only honorable, time-proven ways to success.

Day 192

People whose lives are determined by human flesh focus their minds on matters to do with the flesh, but people whose lives are determined by the spirit focus their minds on matters to do with the spirit. Focus the mind on the flesh, and you'll die; but focus it on the spirit, and you'll have life, and peace.—Romans 8:5–6

Brainy Tip: Our thoughts give our lives meaning—or they can take the meaning away.

Every day scientists are discovering the precise pathways by which changes in human consciousness produce changes in our brains and bodies. Our consciousness—this phenomenal gift from God to be able to think—activates our genes and changes our brains. Science shows that our thoughts, with their embedded feelings, turn sets of genes on and off in complex relationships.

We take facts, experiences, and the events of life and assign meaning to them with our thinking. We may have a fixed set of genes in our chromosomes, but which of those genes are active and how they are active has a great deal to do with how we think and process our experiences. Our thoughts produce words and behaviors, which in turn stimulate more thinking and choices that build more thoughts in an endless cycle. What kind of cycle are you creating with your thoughts? Where is your mind focused? What kind of meaning are you creating in your life? Have you lost your sense of meaning? How so?

Day 193

I will meditate on your precepts, and fix my eyes on your ways.—Psalm 119:15

Brainy Tip: Our thinking determines the quality of our genetic expression, and thus our life.

How we think will determine whether we build health or damage into our brains, because how we think affects the quality of the functionality of our genes. We are naturally designed to focus on the positive, regardless of the emotional allure of information.

However, the freedom of choice we have enables us to consider both good and bad probabilities. If we are lazy and undisciplined in our thinking, we will become reactive and start distorting the reward circuit in our brains, a distortion that affects our genetic function. This leads to temporary highs from the dopamine rush of, for example, gossiping about someone, and if we do this often enough, we will "crave" the high, even though we feel awful mentally and physically afterward. But we are not being controlled by outside influences; we are choosing to focus on the wrong things. Use your mind to fix your thoughts on God's ways and meditate on his precepts, not your selfish desires.

Day 194

So fasten your belts—the belts of your minds! Keep yourselves under control. Set your hope completely on the grace that will be given you when Jesus the Messiah is revealed.—1 Peter 1:13

Brainy Tip: We have the power to discipline our minds, and therefore control our genetic expression, by choosing what we put our hope in.

Science and Scripture both show that we are wired for hope and optimism. When we react by thinking negatively and making negative choices, the quality of our thinking suffers, which means the quality of our brain architecture suffers. When we focus on what is going wrong or what we worry about, our bodies respond to our fears. When we focus on God's life and strength in the midst of difficult times, our bodies respond to our hope and faith. The choice is ours.

Day 195

"What makes someone unclean," he went on, "is what comes out of them."—Mark 7:20

> **Brainy Tip:** Our thoughts can change our DNA, for better or for worse.

Our DNA changes shape according to our thoughts. As you think those negative thoughts about the future—the week ahead, what a person might say or do—even in the absence of the concrete stimulus, that toxic thinking will change your brain wiring in a negative direction and throw your mind and body into stress. This kind of negative thinking puts the body in negative stress, which affects your natural healing capacities. Toxic thinking literally wears down the brain!

Day 196

*But those who wait for the L*ORD *shall renew their strength, they shall mount up with wings like eagles, they shall run and not be weary, they shall walk and not faint.*—Isaiah 40:31

> **Brainy Tip:** The mindset of seeing positive possibilities strengthens and changes the brain and body, while the converse also applies.

An entrepreneurial focus sees multiple possibilities in every situation; it is a mindset that perceives all kinds of probabilities and potentialities. This type of thinking is intrinsically hopeful; you just keep on keeping on till you find success. You appreciate the journey *and* the destination. And the good news is that this is part of the wired-for-love nature of the brain and body—you just have to unlock it! This is something I would spend a lot of time on with my patients, which made a profound difference in their progress.

When you *choose* to develop a mindset that allows you to perceive possibilities, the wired-for-love design of the brain is activated to respond and attempts become possibilities, not failures. This choice is a great predictor of success.

Day 197

Yes: you will be vindicated by your own words—and you will be condemned by your own words.—Matthew 12:37

Brainy Tip: Be aware of what you plant in your mind, because your thoughts are expressed through your words.

What we say and do is based on what we have already built into our minds. We evaluate this information and make our choices based on it, then we choose to build a new thought, and this is what drives what we say or do. We are not driven by forces beyond our conscious control. We are accountable for every thought and decision we make. We are highly intelligent beings with free will, and we are responsible for our choices. If you become more observant of what you say, you gain great insight into your thinking.

Day 198

What's more, my God will meet all your needs, too, out of
his store of glorious riches in King Jesus.—Philippians 4:19

> **Brainy Tip:** Neuroscience shows us how we monitor our own thinking.

One of the exciting features of neuroscientific research is how
the frontal lobes respond when we deliberately and intentionally stand outside ourselves and observe our own thinking.
We can observe our thoughts and actions and make decisions
about them. Suddenly, biblical principles such as "bringing
all thoughts into captivity" or "renewing your mind" become
less difficult when we realize God has given us the equipment
to do these things. This is a glorious richness that God has
built into our design!

Day 199

"I am the true vine," said Jesus, "and my father is the gardener."—John 15:1

Brainy Tip: We are able to observe a situation from a number of different standpoints.

We have what I call the multiple perspective advantage (MPA). I have mentioned this a few times on other days—it is very important because it allows us to develop wisdom.

Our unique, multifaceted nature, made in God's image, allows us to see things from many different angles—many different perspectives. We have the unique opportunity to assess our thoughts and their impact and choose to connect to the vine that is the Messiah. Choosing to connect helps us heal the brain, promote positive growth, and prune off the branches of toxic thinking.

Always take the time to assess each situation from multiple perspectives. Don't shoot yourself in the foot with only one perspective—this bias damages the brain and will lead to unloving words and actions toward others.

Day 200

But you, children, are from God, and you have overcome them, because the one who is in you is greater than the one who is in the world.—1 John 4:4

Brainy Tip: Your brain will follow the instructions and choices of your mind and change its landscape accordingly.

We are directly responsible for what we choose to think about and dwell on, and we make these decisions in the privacy of our own thinking. When we recognize and acknowledge that we need to renew the way we think, speak, and act, it is important to make a distinction between who we truly are and who we have become through toxic choices. Remember, if you wire it in, you can wire it out! You are not a victim of your past. Your brain will follow the instructions and choices of your mind and change its landscape accordingly.

Day 201

The heavens are telling the glory of God; and the firmament proclaims his handiwork.—Psalm 19:1

Brainy Tip: Science is a way of admiring and trusting in God's love for the world.

Science and spirituality are not at loggerheads. Science provides a way of understanding ourselves, our brains and bodies, and the world we live in. It's a glimpse into the magnificence of God—a way of admiring God. The science of thought specifically gives us the "how to" of renewing the mind.

We praise God's grace and greatness when we start seeing the intricacy of how he has made us and constructed the world we live in. This can give us a sense of peace that he is in control and knows what he is doing.

Day 202

So, then, if the spirit of the one who raised Jesus from the dead lives within you, the one who raised the Messiah from the dead will give life to your mortal bodies, too, through his spirit who lives within you.—Romans 8:11

Brainy Tip: You are not a slave to your genes. Genes are not self-emergent, which means they cannot switch themselves on. You switch your genes on with your thinking.

We have been living under a myth called the gene myth, which locates the ultimate power over health and mental wellbeing in the untouchable realm of genes, relegating them to the level of gods. This myth has bound the mental and physical health as well as the peace and happiness of too many people for too long. Almost daily another headline pops up with the highly fashionable concept of a gene for this or a gene for that. You are an alcoholic or are depressed or battle with learning disabilities because you have the gene for alcoholism or depression or learning disabilities or whatever.

It is important to realize that genes can create an environment within us in which a problem may grow, a predisposition or a "curse," but they do not necessarily produce the problem; we can produce it through our choices. The way we react—our thinking and choosing—becomes the signal that activates or deactivates the generational issues in our lives. It is therefore imperative that we ask the Holy Spirit for wisdom regarding our past and every single one of our decisions in the future.

Day 203

What you sow is what you'll reap.—Galatians 6:7

> **Brainy Tip:** Your genes are affected by your choices and experiences.

You control your genes; your genes do not control you. Genes may determine physical characteristics but not psychological phenomena. On the contrary, your genes are constantly being remodeled in response to life experiences.

What kinds of choices, experiences, and reactions are influencing your genes? What are you sowing into your life?

Day 204

What then is faith? It is what gives assurance to our hopes;
it is what gives us conviction about things we can't see.
—Hebrews 11:1

Brainy Tip: We are co-creators of our destiny alongside God.

We are not victims of our biology. We are co-creators of our destiny alongside God. God leads, but we have to choose to let God lead. God has given us the intellect (consciousness or mind) to be co-creators. As such, you have a say in the possible outcomes of your life. You are designed to be in dialogue with God about your life through your intellect.

An analogy I often use to teach this concept is baking a cake. The cake represents a particular life issue you are dealing with. The gift of free will allows us to choose the type of cake we will bake and what we do with this cake. We choose the ingredients and we bake the cake—God doesn't give us the ready-baked cake. We can choose to do this with or without God.

We have been designed to create thoughts, and from these we live out our lives. Whatever you believe in and hope for becomes substance on a physical level, and you act upon this.

Day 205

Yes: if you sow in the field of your flesh you will harvest decay from your flesh, but if you sow in the field of the spirit you will harvest eternal life from the spirit.—Galatians 6:8

Brainy Tip: Through our thoughts, we can be our own brain surgeons.

Our choices—the natural consequences of our thoughts and imagination—get "under the skin" of our DNA and can turn certain genes on and off, changing the structure of the neurons in our brains. Our thoughts, imagination, and choices can change the structure and function of our brains on every level: molecular, genetic, epigenetic, cellular, structural, neurochemical, electromagnetic, and even subatomic. We are literally doing our own brain surgery every moment of every day!

Day 206

So, you see, if the son makes you free, you will be truly free.—John 8:36

> **Brainy Tip:** You are not a victim of your genetic inheritance.

Taken collectively, the studies on epigenetics show us that the good, the bad, and the ugly do come down through the generations, but your mind is the main signal—the epigenetic factor—that switches these genes on or off. You are not destined to live out the negative patterns of your forebearers— you can instead make a life choice to overcome by tweaking their patterns of expression through the way you think. When this sinks in, you will understand what it truly means to be *free*!

Day 207

I'm leaving you peace. I'm giving you my own peace. I don't give gifts in the way the world does. Don't let your hearts be troubled; don't be fearful.—John 14:27

> **Brainy Tip:** Thinking about a problem can transform it into a reality that steals your peace; thinking about a solution can transform it into a reality that will bring you peace.

Epigenetic changes represent a biological response to an environmental signal, the dominant of which is your thought life. That response can be inherited through the generations via the epigenetic marks. But if you remove the signal, the epigenetic marks can begin to fade.

By the same token, if you choose to add a signal—for example, saying something like, "My mother had depression and that's why I have depression, and now my daughter is suffering from depression," then the epigenetic marks can be activated, making this a reality in your life. Constant thinking and speaking about a problem serve as the signal that makes it real, so watch what you think and say.

Day 208

Choose life so that you and your descendants may live.—Deuteronomy 30:19

Brainy Tip: You cannot ignore where you have come from, but you do not have to let it control your life. You can change it.

Your past creates a predisposition, not a destiny. You are not responsible for something you are predisposed to because of ancestral decisions. You are responsible, however, for being aware of these predispositions, evaluating them, and choosing to eliminate them. You are not a victim of what your parents or grandparents have chosen. You are free to choose what kind of life you want to live and the kind of inheritance you want to leave your progeny.

Day 209

When you search for me, you will find me; if you seek me with all your heart.—Jeremiah 29:13

> **Brainy Tip:** The more we seek love with our mind, the more we will experience God's "loveness" in our lives, because this is the default mode of our mind and brain.

Whether we switch on happiness, peace, and good health or switch on anxiety, worry, and negativity, we are changing the physical substance of the brain. Neuroplasticity can operate for us as well as against us, because whatever we think about the most will grow. The more we think about and seek God's love, the more we will discover his powerful love in our own brains, bodies, and lives. Truth and love will always win.

Day 210

When the cares of my heart are many, your consolations cheer my soul.—Psalm 94:19

> **Brainy Tip:** You can reconceptualize toxic thoughts, which means you can get rid of them and redesign a new, healthy way of thinking.

How do you fix toxic thinking? The overriding concept is to apply neuroplasticity in the correct direction by rewiring a negative event or experience with positive thinking. You can consciously choose, preferably under the leading of the Holy Spirit, to bring the memory into consciousness, where it becomes plastic enough to actually be changed. This means the physical substrate of the memory becomes weakened, vulnerable, malleable, and able to be manipulated. You can then choose to replace the crushing mental event with the promises of God. Like an outsider looking in through a window, you can observe the toxic, traumatic memory as a weakening and dying experience and, at the same time, observe the new, healthy experience that is growing. In practicing this daily, you can wire the healthy new thoughts ever more deeply into your brain (see my online programs and books on how to do this). This is renewing the mind in action!

Day 211

*Bless the LORD, O my soul, and do not forget all his benefits—
who forgives all your iniquity, who heals all your diseases,
who redeems your life from the Pit, who crowns you with
steadfast love and mercy, who satisfies you with good as long
as you live so that your youth is renewed like the eagle's.—
Psalm 103:2–5*

Brainy Tip: Changing your thoughts changes the neurons in your brain.

When you choose to focus on God's love, grace, and forgiveness in the midst of dealing with a difficult situation, you change the architecture of your brain. Neurons that don't get enough signal (the constant rehearsing of a negative event) will start firing apart and wiring apart, literally melting away and diminishing the emotion attached to the trauma. In addition, certain chemicals such as oxytocin (which bonds and remolds chemicals), dopamine (which increases focus and attention), and serotonin (which increases feelings of peace and happiness) all start flowing around the traumatic thoughts, weakening them even more. This all helps to disconnect and desynchronize the neurons; if they stop firing together, they will no longer wire together. This leads to wiping out or popping those connections and rebuilding new, healthy ones. Healing is possible!

Day 212

After all, the spirit given to us by God isn't a fearful spirit; it's a spirit of power, love, and prudence.—2 Timothy 1:7

Brainy Tip: You have the ability to operate with power, making your mind and brain work for you and not against you.

Everyone seems to be talking about mindfulness and taking the time to invest in yourself. But how do you really make your mind work for you? How do you use your mind to shape your life? How do you "invest" in yourself, creating a lifestyle that promotes both brain and body health? How do you go beyond awareness of, calming down, and acknowledging feelings, thoughts, and bodily sensations in the present moment to making sustainable long-lasting changes?

You can use the power of your mind to think, feel, and choose in your Perfect You—your customized mode of thinking! Don't let the media, doctors, or other people in your life tell you otherwise. You have the power in your unique mind to change the negative, toxic manifestations in your life and embrace your Perfect You.

Day 213

Beloved, I pray that all is going well with you, and that you are every bit as healthy physically as you are spiritually.—3 John 2

> **Brainy Tip:** Our perspective is incredibly important.

We need to recognize that neither society nor our brains determine what we do with our lives. We need to recognize that our *own* thoughts—with our own unique perspectives—can hinder our ability to think, learn, and succeed beyond the limits of any society. Have you ever scrolled through Instagram, paralyzed by the feeling that your life somehow doesn't "measure up"? Have you ever felt swamped at work, with a crazy *Devil Wears Prada*–style boss shouting down at you in an endless, meaningless cycle, because you felt that was the kind of job a responsible adult had to have and this was what you were supposed to do? Have you ever felt lost preparing for an exam you knew you were going to fail? Sometimes we can be our own worst enemy.

Our perception of our environment, plus how we manage our environment and what is going on in our lives, influences the functionality of our brains and bodies. If you change your perception, you change your biology and your environment. You become the master of your life instead of a victim.

Action on both a spiritual and biological level is required for true, lasting change to take place.

Day 214

But when the kindness and generous love of God our savior appeared, he saved us, not by works that we did in righteousness, but in accordance with his own mercy, through the washing of the new birth and the renewal of the holy spirit, which was poured out richly upon us through Jesus, our king and savior, so that we might be justified by his grace and be made his heirs, in accordance with the hope of the life of the age to come. —Titus 3:4–7

Brainy Tip: The mind controls the brain.

The world may tell us that the mind is what the brain does, but God shows us, through Scripture and science, that the brain will do what the mind tells it to do. When your spirit, under the leading of the Holy Spirit, directs your mind, then the gold standard of thinking is achieved. You *can* move from survival to success—it all begins in your mind. Recognizing both the impact of your sociocultural context and your own thoughts, you can redefine your past, reimagine your present, and realize your future.

Day 215

Bad company kills off good habits!—1 Corinthians 15:33

> **Brainy Tip:** Your environment influences your thoughts, words, and actions.

How you live, the cultural environment you live in, whatever you immerse yourself in, your beliefs and the beliefs of those around you, how you interact with those people, your faith and how you grow it, what you expose yourself to—all of these lead to differences in the way you focus your attention and have a direct effect on how your proteins are synthesized, how your enzymes act, and how your neurochemicals work together. They affect the architecture of your brain, thereby influencing what you think, what you say, and what you do.

Day 216

We also celebrate in our sufferings, because we know that suffering produces patience, patience produces a well-formed character, and a character like that produces hope. Hope, in its turn, does not make us ashamed, because the love of God has been poured out in our hearts through the holy spirit who has been given to us.—Romans 5:3–5

Brainy Tip: You cannot change your thinking overnight.

Doing your own brain surgery or neuroplastic intervention of toxic thinking and renewing your mind is based on regular exercising of your brain. True, lasting change takes place over time through *continual* persistence. There is no quick fix, pill, or magic trick that can change the way you think, speak, and act over time. Persistence and discipline are the keys to a renewed way of thinking, which changes the brain physically, chemically, structurally, and functionally. If you are looking for a quick fix, you will be disappointed. God helps us as much as we help ourselves. We have to take the first step; we have to make that first decision.

Day 217

Don't let evil conquer you. Rather, conquer evil with good.
—Romans 12:21

> **Brainy Tip:** We control what we allow to influence the way we live our lives.

Since psychosocial factors modulate the course of certain diseases—such as cardiovascular disease, diabetes, and asthma—this means the things going on in the environment get into the mind, changing the brain and having an impact on the body. Understanding how God designed neuroplasticity to work for and against us will help us move forward and succeed in life by controlling what we allow into our minds, thereby controlling what we allow to influence the way we live our lives.

Day 218

Be still, and know that I am God!—Psalm 46:10

Brainy Tip: Quiet time is necessary for your mental and physical health.

The ability to quiet your mind, focus your attention on the present issue, capture your thoughts, and dismiss the distractions that come your way is an excellent and powerful skill that God has placed within you. In the busy age we live in, however, we have trained ourselves out of this natural and necessary ability. Natural because it is wired into the design of the brain, allowing the brain to capture and discipline chaotic rogue thoughts; necessary because it calms our spirits so we can tune in and listen to God. It is therefore incredibly important that we incorporate quiet time into our lives— periods when we can just be still, think, and praise God.

Day 219

Cast your burden on the LORD, and he will sustain you; he will never permit the righteous to be moved.—Psalm 55:22

Brainy Tip: When you choose to operate in love, you increase your sustainability and resilience during tough situations.

Think of your mind as the movement of information as energy through your nervous system. Each thought has quantum energy, and electrochemical and electromagnetic signals that flow largely below your level of awareness. Just thinking about a loved one, for example, can cause positive structural changes in the caudate nucleus of the brain, which is closely linked to feelings of reward and happiness. Likewise, healthy electromagnetic signals and quantum fields fire up in response to a good attitude, giving you strength to face the day.

The converse also applies. Stress, which can be good for you, can become incredibly toxic, depending on your perception of a situation. The other day, a friend was telling me how just driving past her previous workplace brought back a significant physical heart pain, which she used to experience daily in the toxic work environment. Her symptoms had disappeared once she resigned. The treatment in this case wasn't medication or surgery, it was the self-care decision to get another job! She chose to love her health over her toxic, stressful job.

We need sustainability to cope with life, and the good news is that you come with a built-in sustainability system that is activated when you renew your mind and act in love!

Day 220

But their delight is in the law of the LORD, and on his law they meditate day and night.—Psalm 1:2

Brainy Tip: Healthy deep thinking leads to a healthy life.

Research has shown that five to sixteen minutes a day of focused, intense capturing of thoughts shifts frontal brain states to function at higher levels and can help you to engage with the world wisely. Those same five to sixteen minutes of intense, deep thinking activity increase the chances of a happier outlook on life! Thinking deeply about healthy thoughts and intellectually challenging information is essential for a good, healthy life.

Day 221

Every creation of God, you see, is good.—1 Timothy 4:4

> **Brainy Tip:** The brain is designed to reflect the glory of God.

God's order is clearly reflected in the organization of the brain. God has designed the brain to work in a series of coordinated networks—his creation is always "good." The scientific expression for this is "integrative functional organization," which basically means that all parts of the brain are connected, work together, and impact each other, just as all the parts of the kingdom are designed to work for the glory of God. But this only happens when we think correctly in "loveness" (there's that weird word again)! "Loveness" is thinking God's thoughts after him. It is about embracing the goodness of creation that is inside you and reflecting this goodness into the world. What does love look like in your life?

Day 222

"What makes someone unclean," he went on, "is what comes out of them. Evil intentions come from inside, out of people's hearts. . . . They are what make someone unclean."
—*Mark 7:20–23*

> **Brainy Tip:** Research shows that the signals of the mind, which are considered nonphysical light waves or packets of energy, form 90 to 99 percent of who we are.

We cannot ignore the intangible, powerful mind element of who we are. As thoughts travel through our brains at quantum speeds, neurons fire together in distinctive ways, and those patterns of activity transform our neural structure. Essentially, the way you think, through the mindsets you adopt, will influence the neural correlates in your brain, thereby influencing your words and actions. In turn, these words and actions influence the brain, and a feedback loop is established based on this mindset. A feedback loop can be changed at any time through your *choice* to alter your mindset—what is in your heart.

God has designed the brain in such a way that the intrinsic activity in the nonconscious part of our minds is where most of the mind-action takes place. It is where we are thinking, choosing, building, and sorting thoughts. It is the constant, high-energy activity that is always going on in the nonconscious mind, even when we are resting. What we consciously think and what we say and do are all driven by the activity in the nonconscious mind. The nonconscious mind has the roots of all our words and actions, and we choose with our minds what these roots will be—it is our "heart" or inner person.

Day 223

"The sabbath was made for humans," he said, "not humans for the sabbath."—Mark 2:27

Brainy Tip: We are designed to rest.

When we go into a directed rest—a focused, introspective state—we enhance and increase the effectiveness of the activity in the nonconscious mind. We do not stop all activity, just as God did not rest in the modern sense (that is, cease working) in the creation accounts but rather established his rule in the temple after a period of creative activity.[1] By giving ourselves time to think in a directed rest state, we increase the gamma waves in our brain, which are involved in attention, memory building, and learning, and increase brain activity linked to positive emotions like happiness. PET scans as well as EEG and qEEG recordings show portions of the brain bulk up that produce happiness, wisdom, and peace.

Day 224

Everyone who is called by my name, whom I created for my glory, whom I formed and made.—Isaiah 43:7

Brainy Tip: Choosing to shift from a threat mindset to an opportunity mindset changes the way we function.

God's glorious love is manifested through each of us. When we see a threat as an opportunity, we are, in essence, reflecting God's glory. You have so much power in you to thrive instead of strive. When you consciously choose to practice operating in a mindset of gratitude, for instance, you will get a surge of rewarding neurotransmitters such as dopamine and experience both a general sense of being alert and a brightening of the mind.

The path to success is directly linked to reflecting God's glory, and it starts with your thinking—your brain and your life will respond accordingly.

How will the world understand the glory of God unless you and I step up into our Perfect You, the unique piece of God's glory for which we were made?

Day 225

The purpose of all this is so that you may run away from the corruption of lust that is in the world, and may become partakers of the divine nature. So, because of this, you should strain every nerve to supplement your faith with virtue, and your virtue with knowledge, and your knowledge with self-control, and your self-control with patience, and your patience with piety, and your piety with family affection, and your family affection with love.—2 Peter 1:4–7

Brainy Tip: We have to control what we think if we want to speak and act in love.

An undisciplined mind is filled with a continuous stream of worries, fears, and distorted perceptions that trigger degenerative processes in the mind and body. We cannot afford not to bring all thoughts into captivity to the Messiah. Catching our thoughts is necessary because it calms our spirits so we can tune in and listen to God and live according to his love—we can "[partake in] the divine nature" of God.

Day 226

I will meditate on your precepts, and fix my eyes on your ways. I will delight in your statutes; I will not forget your word.—Psalm 119:15–16

Brainy Tip: Reconceptualizing toxic thoughts requires being aware of them in the first place—awareness weakens them so they become susceptible to change.

When your mind is busy with intrinsic activity (directed rest) such as introspection, meditating on the Bible, thinking things through, letting your mind wander, sleeping, and deep thinking (even under anesthetic!), there is a constant chatter between the networks of the brain in the nonconscious mind.

Taking the time to think and meditate on what is good and not just react impulsively to the circumstances of life really gets your brain working in the right way. Indeed, when we have flexible and creative thinking, we are able to shift between thoughts and capture and control thoughts. We should be practicing this continually throughout the day, every day!

Day 227

Those of steadfast mind you keep in peace—in peace because they trust in you.—Isaiah 26:3

> **Brainy Tip:** Mental flexibility allows us to control our reactions to the circumstances of life, which brings peace.

We need mental flexibility as we go through life. It is always worth reminding ourselves that we cannot control the events and circumstances of life but we can control our reactions to those events and circumstances. Controlling our reactions requires flexibility in our thinking, which is built into the design of the brain. God has literally crafted our brains to work for us and not to control us, and his peace guards our minds so that we can think well!

Day 228

Draw near to God, and he will draw near to you.—James 4:8

Brainy Tip: Moments of peace and quiet help us tap into and develop wisdom.

When we shift into our default mode network (DMN) during times when we are still and meditate, we don't switch off to rest and go mentally blank. Quite the contrary; we switch off in order to switch on a mode of thinking that gives us perspective, wisdom, and the opportunity to connect with God. This is a state of mind in which we switch off to the external and switch on to the internal.

Do this as often as you can, on a daily basis, and watch your thought life improve!

Day 229

I'm leaving you peace. I'm giving you my own peace. I don't give gifts in the way the world does. Don't let your hearts be troubled; don't be fearful.—John 14:27

Brainy Tip: Through deep, intellectual thinking and meditation, we can connect to the spiritual part of who we are.

In a deeply intellectual state, involved networks remain active and the shifting between them also remains active, but it is a different kind of activity. It is more focused and introspective. So when our brain enters the rest circuit (DMN), we don't actually rest; we move into a highly intelligent, self-reflective, directed state. And the more often we go there, the more we get in touch with the deep, spiritual part of who we are. I believe God has created this state to directly connect us to the Holy Spirit and to help us develop and practice an awareness of his presence—we get in a rhythm with the Spirit.

Day 230

So God blessed the seventh day and hallowed it, because on it God rested from all the work that he had done in creation.—Genesis 2:3

Brainy Tip: Our brain needs periods of directed rest.

The DMN is a primary network that we switch into when we switch off from the outside world and move into a state of focused and deliberate deep thinking. It activates to even higher levels when a person is daydreaming, introspecting, or letting his or her mind wander in an organized, exploratory way through the endless myriad of thoughts within it. It's a directed, deeply intellectual state that focuses inward and tunes out the outside world. It is a cessation from the active, external demands of the world, in order that we can focus on the immense creative and imaginative power in our minds.

A Sabbath is therefore not just "switching off" in the modern sense, which in itself has physical and mental health benefits, nor is it simply taking a rest on Sundays. It is a way to tap into, harness, and discover the immense potential of the human mind—potential that has the power to bring heaven to earth and change the world. It is a period of restoration and renewal, a period after all the battles have been won; this type of Sabbath brings order and balance to life.[1] This type of rest is essential to our mental and physical wellbeing.

Day 231

"The sabbath was made for humans," he said, "not humans for the sabbath."—Mark 2:27

Brainy Tip: Switching off to external influences helps us discipline our minds.

Regular deep thinkers—by this I mean those who have adopted a disciplined, focused, and reflective thought life in which they bring all thoughts into captivity—show that their DMN is more active and that there is more switching back and forth between the networks in their brains. This means their brains are more active, growing more branches, and integrating and linking more thoughts, which translates into increased intelligence and wisdom and that wonderful feeling of peace.

Day 232

That's why I'm telling you, everything that you request in prayer, everything you ask God for, believe that you receive it, and it will happen for you.—Mark 11:24

Brainy Tip: Deep, intellectual thinking helps us connect with our source and renew our mind.

When we pray, when we catch our thoughts, when we memorize and quote Scriptures, when we study new knowledge with the attempt to understand it, we move into a deep meditative state. This great state of mind is also activated when we intellectualize deeply about information—perhaps what we are studying or a skill we are developing in our job or in our life. We are highly intellectual beings created to have relationship with a highly intellectual God. We should never underestimate how brilliant we are. We are only limited by how we see ourselves.

Day 233

For you, O Lord, are good and forgiving, abounding in stead-fast love to all who call on you.—Psalm 86:5

> **Brainy Tip:** We can retrain the brain to focus on the good things in life.

We step into our "normal" when we are grateful for the stead-fast mercy and love of God, because we are wired for his love. We retrain the brain, tapping into our natural optimism bias. Having an "attitude of gratitude," so to speak, enables us to see more possibility, feel more energy, and succeed at higher levels in our lives.

I emphasize *retrain* the brain as opposed to *train* the brain. It is incorrect to assume that the brain has a negative bias and that we have to fight off its natural tendency to scan for and spot the undesirable. This kind of negative mindset will actually work against the natural optimism bias of brain function and upset thinking patterns!

Our minds need time to understand what our spirits al-ready know and how we can use this knowledge to change our lives and the world for God's glory.

Day 234

"Martha, Martha," he replied, "you are fretting and fussing about so many things. Only one thing matters. Mary has chosen the best part, and it's not going to be taken away from her."—Luke 10:41–42

Brainy Tip: "Hurry sickness" can create chaos in the brain.

In the busyness of life and the flurry of everyday activity, we expose ourselves to the possibility of developing a chaotic mindset with the net result of neurochemical and electromagnetic chaos in the brain. This feels like endless loops and spirals of thinking that can easily get out of control.

When we activate the DMN, however, it is almost like a Sabbath in the brain, which is a cessation from the conscious flurry of work and a withdrawal into the depths of our magnificent minds. It is like a mental rebooting process to reconnect with who we are and with our Messiah, enabling us to bring perspective to the issues of life. It stimulates, rather than halts, our productivity.

Day 235

Are you having a real struggle? Come to me! Are you carrying a big load on your back? Come to me—I'll give you a rest!—Matthew 11:28

> **Brainy Tip:** Constant work can affect our mental health. The brain needs time to rest and reboot.

When we don't engage in a disciplined and focused self-reflective pattern of thinking that activates the DMN, we may experience negative self-esteem, get stuck, be unable to cope, and have a tendency to focus on the problem and not the solution. In fact, as things go wrong in the processing of information, the mishandled data is passed on to other networks in the brain, where it creates additional problems. These additional problems can be experienced as memory issues, fuzzy thinking, anxiety, depression, and many other manifestations, including neuropsychiatric disorders.

In my experience, helping my patients analyze and write down their thoughts in a self-reflective way during these "thinker" moments, when they were potentially ruminating on negative situations and getting stuck, was an effective way to develop their imagination. When they could work out which thoughts were free-flowing and track their direction over time, as well as which thoughts were getting stuck, they could also evaluate if these thoughts were giving them a sense of peace or disturbing their minds. Then they could look for an alternate way of thinking, and I would teach them to practice developing the newly reconceptualized positive thoughts, automatizing them over time into helpful, useful, and successful memories.

Day 236

Just as the body without the spirit is dead, you see, so faith without works is dead.—James 2:26

Brainy Tip: Good thinking will lead to good actions.

The task positive network (TPN) supports the active thinking required for making decisions. As we focus our thinking and activate the DMN, at some point in our thinking process we move into active decision-making. This activates the TPN, and we experience this as action. Action completes the cycle of building up and breaking down thoughts.

Think of ways you can incorporate this action into your daily schedule to affect positive changes in your life.

Day 237

Can any of you add fifteen inches to your height just by worrying about it?—Matthew 6:27

Brainy Tip: Negative thinking affects our ability to think clearly.

Toxic negative thinking produces increased activity in the DMN and decreased activity in the TPN. This results in maladaptive, depressive ruminations and a decrease in the ability to solve problems. This makes us feel foggy, confused, negative, and depressed. Negative thinking decreases our wisdom and clarity!

Day 238

For where there is jealousy and contention, there you will get
unruly behavior and every kind of evil practice. —James 3:16

Brainy Tip: Bad thinking habits lead to bad behavior.

God is a God of order and balance, and he has fashioned
our spirit, soul, and body this way. It is quite simple: when
we don't follow his ordinances, there will be consequences.
The brain moves into an unbalanced state, producing neurochemical and electromagnetic chaos.

We need downtime to function optimally. To cope with
the demands of life, our minds and brains need to internally
reboot, which can only happen when we are alone with our
thoughts. We literally need to switch off all external stimuli,
giving our thoughts some quality "me time."

It is incredibly important that we learn to be still and enjoy
the present. We need to learn to savor the pleasure of "now"
and not just marinate in the misery of the past or imagine that
the grass will be greener in the future. The satisfaction that
comes from being truly happy plays a vital role in success.

Day 239

Anxiety weighs down the human heart.—Proverbs 12:25

Brainy Tip: Brooding can affect our mental health.

When rumination turns into unproductive brooding and negative issues are blown out of proportion, it is detrimental to the brain and to good life choices. When this happens, introspection activating the DMN turns from a healthy coping-and-solution focus to an unhealthy passive-and-maladaptive focus, which can result in worrying, anxiety, and depression.

Day 240

He must be hospitable, a lover of goodness, sensible, just, holy, and self-controlled.—Titus 1:8

Brainy Tip: Disciplining your thoughts leads to a sensible and self-controlled mental life.

Through modifying your mental practices toward a more disciplined, focused, and reflective thought life, you can build up healthy neural real estate in the brain that helps you bring your thoughts into captivity and deal with the demands of today's modern world.

Your mind can powerfully and unexpectedly change your brain in positive ways when you intentionally direct your attention! The ability to think about, process, and maintain a balanced lifestyle should therefore always be a top priority when it comes to coping with what life throws at you. "Thinker" moments should be an integral part of your mental self-care regimen. The brain needs "thinker" time for its health and functioning, including the prevention of dementias!

Remember, the most efficient way to improve your brain is a daily step-by-step process—a *lifestyle* of thinking your brain into better functioning.

Day 241

Let your eyes look directly forward, and your gaze be straight before you. Keep straight the path of your feet, and all your ways will be sure.—Proverbs 4:25–26

Brainy Tip: Focused attention is one of the keys to a successful life.

One of the plagues of modern existence is multitasking, which leads to the further plagues of "hurry sickness" and obsessive time management. The truth about multitasking is that it is a persistent myth. What we really do is shift our attention rapidly from task to task, resulting in two bad things: (1) we don't devote as much focused attention as we should to a specific activity, task, or piece of information, and (2) we sacrifice the quality of our attention. I call this "milkshake-multitasking." This poor focusing of attention and lack of quality in our thought lives is the complete opposite of how the brain is designed to function and causes a level of brain damage. Every rapid, incomplete, and poor-quality shift of thought is like making a milkshake with your brain cells and neurochemicals. Hence it is extremely important to choose to focus your full attention on one task at a time if you want to see your performance and your peace improve!

251

Day 242

My child, be attentive to my words; incline your ear to my sayings. Do not let them escape from your sight; keep them within your heart. For they are life to those who find them, and healing to all their flesh.—Proverbs 4:20–22

Brainy Tip: Deep, focused attention positively affects our mental and physical health.

What does deep, focused, intellectual attention look like versus milkshake-multitasking? The answer is modeled in Proverbs 4:20–22: listening, concentrating, and meditating on what you hear and observe. It is very interesting that every cell in the body is connected to the heart—and the brain controls the heart and the mind controls the brain. Remember, whatever we are thinking about affects every cell in our body. When we operate in "loveness," our life flourishes.

Day 243

These are the things you should think through: whatever is true, whatever is holy, whatever is upright, whatever is pure, whatever is attractive, whatever has a good reputation; anything virtuous, anything praiseworthy.—Philippians 4:8

Brainy Tip: We can only truly focus on one thing at a time. What are you focusing on?

Today, so much attention is paid to Twitter, Instagram, and Facebook that we often forget to enjoy the moment. We are told by so-called social media experts that information needs to be in bite-sized amounts and in a constant stream. This is not stimulation; it is bombardment. We have been reduced to 140 characters and an addiction to looking for the next informational high. Many of us cannot just sit quietly and enjoy reading a book, allowing our imagination to take flight.

Of course, social media plays an important role in society, business, and life. When used correctly and in a balanced way, it is a phenomenal communications tool—I am all for progress. Used incorrectly and obsessively, however, this good thing becomes a bad thing. Social media has become as ubiquitous as television in our everyday lives, and research shows that multitasking social media can be as addictive as drugs, alcohol, and chemical substance abuse. It can easily become our idol as we give our social media accounts more and more attention with our minds, meditating on Twitter rather than using our minds to think deeply about what is good, upright, just, and holy.

Day 244

The heart of our God is full of mercy; that's why his daylight has dawned from on high, bringing light to the dark, as we sat in death's shadow, guiding our feet in the path of peace.—Luke 1:78–79

Brainy Tip: Milkshake-multitasking affects our ability to be at peace.

Life is all about balance. Our brain responds with healthy patterns, circuits, and neurochemicals when we think deeply, but not when we skim only the surface of multiple pieces of information. Research actually shows that people who think they are handling multitasking well are actually reducing their intelligence!

The peace that comes from God helps us think, choose, decide, and settle the questions and problems that arise in our life—it is a guiding force in our lives. But milkshake-multitasking switches on confusion in our brains, making this type of mental harmony impossible.

Day 245

Fools despise wisdom and instruction.—Proverbs 1:7

Brainy Tip: Uncontrolled thinking habits lead to foolish decisions.

Milkshake-multitasking decreases our attention, making us decreasingly able to focus on our thought habits. This opens us up to shallow and weak judgments and decisions and results in passive mindlessness. Deep, intellectual thought, however, results in interactive mindfulness that leads to the next step of deep thinking, which in turn requires engaging passionately with the world. We need to increase our awareness of our thoughts and take the time to understand and reflect on them if we truly want to reflect God's glory into our communities and bring heaven to earth.

Day 246

The hope of the righteous ends in gladness.—Proverbs 10:28

Brainy Tip: Thinking deeply improves brain health.

Taking the time to think deeply and carefully can improve focus, concentration, understanding, efficiency, and overall effectiveness in producing quality work. It can also result in positive emotional changes, specifically in self-motivation and self-esteem. Over time, deep thinking can improve overall cognitive and emotional functioning. Once someone is set on a healthy thinking path, the benefits of a healthy thought life can continue upward in a developing fashion!

Day 247

But as for you, keep your balance in everything! Put up with suffering; do the work of an evangelist; complete the particular task assigned to you.—2 Timothy 4:5

> **Brainy Tip:** When you learn how to harness the power of your mind, you set yourself on the road to success.

Deep, intellectual thinking activates the prefrontal cortex (just above your eyebrows) in a positive way, resulting in increased concentration, less distraction, less switching between tasks, more effective switching between tasks, decreased emotional volatility, and overall increase in job completion. This type of intentional thinking can also improve connections within and between nerve networks, specifically in the front part of the brain and between the front and middle parts of the brain. In sum, if you want to succeed in life, you need to learn how to use your ability to think!

Day 248

So, now, faith, hope, and love remain.—1 Corinthians 13:13

Brainy Tip: Faith, hope, and love change the brain for the better.

To think positively about our prospects, we must be able to imagine ourselves in the future. Our brains may have stamps from the past, but they are being rewired by our expectation of the future. Imagining a positive future reduces the pain of the past. Faith in God's promises and his love for us motivates us to pursue these goals. Hope leads to expectation, which creates peace, excitement, and health in our minds, thus increasing brain and body health.

Day 249

Take my instruction instead of silver, and knowledge rather than choice gold; for wisdom is better than jewels, and all that you may desire cannot compare with her.—Proverbs 8:10–11

Brainy Tip: Deliberate thinking leads to knowledge and wisdom.

Deep, intentional thinking increases gyrification, a lovely word that means more folds in the cortex of the brain. These extra folds allow the brain to process information faster, make decisions quicker, and improve memory. Deep thinking is therefore an essential component of knowledge and wisdom!

Day 250

For wisdom will come into your heart, and knowledge will be pleasant to your soul.—Proverbs 2:10

> **Brainy Tip:** Controlling your thought life will help you maintain your peace and joy.

When we take our thoughts captive and discipline our thinking, positive physical brain changes occur. These changes allow us to embrace our wired-for-love design, helping us truly live out the kind of life God wants us to live. Consciously controlling our thought life means that we do not allow thoughts to run rampant through our minds. Instead, we learn to engage interactively with each thought, taking control over and learning to enjoy the moment we are in. Essentially, our job is to analyze a thought before we decide either to accept or reject it.

We are better able to love ourselves as we recognize our powerful ability to think and choose, we are better able to love others as we recognize the same incredible power in them, and we are better able to love the world as we understand how we have the ability to change it for the better.

Day 251

My people are destroyed for lack of knowledge. —Hosea 4:6

Brainy Tip: Failing to recognize the power in our minds can have negative health effects.

When we learn to take our thoughts captive and renew our minds, we grow in our understanding, which results in positive structural changes in our brain that benefit our mental and physical health. On the other hand, if we allow our minds to wander and ruminate on our fears, concerns, and problems, our brain responds by changing in a negative direction, which can negatively affect our mental and physical health, bringing illness and death into our lives.

Day 252

Think back to your own call, my brothers and sisters. Not many of you were wise in human terms. Not many of you were powerful. Not many were nobly born. But God chose the foolish things of the world to shame the wise; God chose the weak things of the world to shame the strong; God chose the insignificant and despised things of the world— yes, even things that don't exist!—to abolish the power of the things that do exist.—1 Corinthians 1:26–28

Brainy Tip: The more we feel like we are failures, the more likely we are to fail.

We need to recognize that society alone is not the sole factor in determining what we do with our lives. Our own thoughts can hinder our ability to think, learn, and succeed beyond the limits of any society. Have you ever scrolled through Instagram, paralyzed by the feeling that your life somehow doesn't measure up? Have you ever felt swamped at work or stuck in an endless, meaningless cycle of nine-to-five? Have you ever felt lost preparing for an exam you knew you were going to fail? Sometimes we can be our own worst enemy!

We need to remember that often the people who change the world come from unexpected places. We need to remember that where we fall short, God steps in. And we need to remember that success is subjective. You can only be as successful as *you*, not as successful as someone else. And you are as successful as you want to be.

Day 253

He gave five talents to the first, two to the next, and one to the last—each according to his ability.—Matthew 25:15

> **Brainy Tip:** What we choose to think about impacts how we use our time.

Our thoughts can either limit us to what we believe we can do or free us to develop abilities well beyond our expectations or the expectations of others. When we choose a mindset that extends our abilities rather than limits them, we will experience greater intellectual satisfaction, emotional control, and mental and physical health.

But nothing worthwhile happens in an instant. We can turn dreams into realities, but first we have to realize that it takes longer than the average one-second lifespan of a Twitter post to make a change. The technological age has brought with it a desire to see things, including change and success, as instantaneous. Yet there is no quick fix to success in school, work, and life. Trying to make things happen fast and then giving up when they do not happen at the speed you have become accustomed to is unhealthy. It can cause you anguish and put your brain and body into toxic stress, keeping you stuck in a toxic cycle—a cycle you can end any time you choose to end it.

We have been given "talents," and they take time to develop. We have something unique and wonderful to give to the world. We *choose* what we do with what we have been given. And we will be held responsible for how we use it.

Day 254

I want them to experience all the wealth of definite under-standing, and to come to the knowledge of God's mystery—the Messiah, the king!—Colossians 2:2

Brainy Tip: When you learn to think with understanding, you learn to live the good life.

Activating your brain through good choices allows it to build successful, meaningful memory that enables you to live a successful, meaningful life. As when you train your body for a marathon or a new exercise in the gym, your brain needs time to develop and achieve success, and you do this training of your brain with your mind.

We readily accept that it takes time to develop skill and expertise in a sport, yet when it comes to the mind, this wisdom often seems to disappear from our mental logic. Such a mindset leads to an endless cycle of cram learning for an exam or for something needed for work and then forgetting most of it the next day. Don't get stuck on this treadmill! Take charge and take the time to develop the wealth of wisdom you have in your brain.

Day 255

Like living stones yourselves, you are being built up into a spiritual house, to be a holy priesthood, to offer spiritual sacrifices that will be well pleasing to God through Jesus the Messiah.—1 Peter 2:5

Brainy Tip: Deep thinking to understand allows us to change our world for the better.

In order for a memory to be usable, it needs lots of energy, which it gets when we attempt to understand information. A memory gets lots of "packets" of energy (quanta) when you repeatedly think about a memory in different ways on a daily basis, which results in the required neurochemical and structural changes in the brain that make this memory a usable and useful thought. A useful memory, therefore, has lots of energy, making it *accessible*. When a memory becomes accessible, it informs the next decision, such as informing the answer on an exam or the solution to an issue. If you do not automatize the memory, however, it will not be accessible and therefore not helpful to you. In order to turn long-term memory into habits, you will have to choose the *hard work* route of investing time in your thought life.

Unfortunately, most people give up within the first week of learning and do not push through. As a result, they have to start all over again, which is not only tedious and disheartening but also creates negative feedback loops. Quick fixes and memory tricks are illusions—do not let them fool you. We are the high priesthood of creation. We need to think, and hence live, in such a way that reflects our vocation as stewards of the world.

Day 256

Before I formed you in the womb I knew you, and before you were born I consecrated you.—Jeremiah 1:5

Brainy Tip: No one can compare to you.

Regardless of what you or anyone you know has told you, you can learn. You can succeed at life. When you learn how to learn—exploring, understanding, and mastering the art of mental self-care—you can go beyond mindfulness, developing a whole-mind lifestyle that allows you to transform your neighborhood, your community, your nation, and your world. Remember, who you are is brilliant, exciting, and inspiring, because you are made in the image of a brilliant, exciting, and inspiring God. Do not let anyone or anything make you think you are less than what you are.

Day 257

But the LORD said to Samuel, "Do not look on his appearance or on the height of his stature, because I have rejected him; for the LORD does not see as mortals see; they look on the outward appearance, but the LORD looks on the heart."—1 Samuel 16:7

Brainy Tip: How you see the world affects how you live in the world.

Your mind can unlock your ability to think, learn, and succeed beyond what you can imagine. Your success, however, depends on your mindset. Mindsets are ways of thinking about specific tasks; they underscore the power your mind has to change the physical structure of your brain. They are the lens that shapes the way you see and interact with the world. They are essential to mental self-care, since they impact the way you think, speak, and act. What kind of mindsets do you have? Are they holding you back or propelling you forward? What do you see when you look at your life, at other people, or at the world?

Day 258

May the God of hope fill you with all joy and peace in believing, so that you may overflow with hope by the power of the holy spirit.—Romans 15:13

Brainy Tip: You have the power to change toxic mindsets every ten seconds.

Your brain is finely attuned to your mind; it is designed to respond to your conscious thinking every ten seconds. This literally means you can consciously evaluate what you are thinking about more or less six times a minute, which also means you can talk to the Spirit of God about six times a minute! You can be filled with joy, peace, hope, and power every ten seconds, which can dramatically affect the way you live your life for the better.

Day 259

Happy are those who do not follow the advice of the wicked, or take the path that sinners tread, or sit in the seat of scoffers; but their delight is in the law of the LORD, and on his law they meditate day and night. They are like trees planted by streams of water, which yield their fruit in its season, and their leaves do not wither. In all that they do, they prosper.—Psalm 1:1–3

Brainy Tip: Success starts with a healthy mindset.

Every moment of every day, your brain and body are physically reacting and changing in response to the thoughts that run through your mind. Your mindsets add "flavor" to these thoughts, making your brain and body work for you or against you. Understanding how mindsets form and how they change your thinking is a practical and helpful way to understand the power of your mind to change your brain. Mindsets help you see the power of your perceptions while optimizing your thought life by generating the correct perceptions, revealing your inner strength and resilience. The correct mindsets are integral to succeeding in school, work, and life, because they allow you to see and experience the world in a different and more dynamic way.

Day 260

A glad heart makes a cheerful countenance, but by sorrow of heart the spirit is broken.—Proverbs 15:13

Brainy Tip: You are as happy, healthy, and successful as you want to be.

On day 258 you learned that you can communicate with the Spirit of God every ten seconds—amazing! The nonconscious mind is even faster, operating at about four hundred billion actions per second, and *you control* what you put into your nonconscious mind.

The thoughts we build into the nonconscious mind have the potential to improve our peace, health, vision, fitness, strength, and much more, because these thoughts form the basis of our mindsets and worldview. The ability to think, feel, and choose and build thoughts into mindsets is one of the most powerful things in the universe, because this power is the source of all human creativity and imagination.

Remember, your life follows the direction of your mind, and your mind follows the direction of your choices.

Day 261

[There is] a time to weep, and a time to laugh; a time to mourn, and a time to dance.—Ecclesiastes 3:4

Brainy Tip: Being satisfied about where you are in life is as important as dreaming of the future.

Dreaming about the future is important for our mental health, giving us a sense of hope, yet we also need to learn to enjoy the journey of life moment by moment. We need to learn to savor the pleasure of "now," and not just marinate in the misery of the past or imagine that the grass will be greener in the future. When we choose to truly tune in to the "now," to see, listen, feel, move, taste, and inhale the present, using all our senses to soak up the minute beauty of the moment, we enhance our thinking, thereby enhancing our ability to learn and succeed at life.

Day 262

The plans of the diligent lead surely to abundance, but everyone who is hasty comes only to want.—Proverbs 21:5

Brainy Tip: Your brain responds to organizing and planning.

You can turn dreams into realities, but first you have to have a plan. That plan comes from your Perfect You thinking. Instead of trying to think like Einstein, you need to think like *you*.

We should recognize that Albert Einstein embraced his own unique way of thinking about and interacting with the world. His gift of thinking allowed him to develop his memory and release his genius, transforming the world of science. Who knows what you can achieve when you think and learn in your customized, excellent way? You would make a lousy Einstein, but you make a great you! You need to realize that you are wonderful just the way you are. We need to recognize the genius in ourselves as well as in each other—this is a journey that takes a lifetime, so learn to enjoy the ride!

Day 263

For you are all children of God, through faith, in the Messiah, Jesus.—Galatians 3:26

Brainy Tip: Different is not a value judgment.

Different doesn't have to mean misunderstood. We don't have to live life frustrated, upset, and discouraged by strained relationships. Just as you can renew your mind and create healthy thought patterns, you can grow and develop insight and understanding that will lead to peace, respect, and love in all of your relationships. In other words, we need each other. We complement each other in every setting—the office, the community, the classroom, the courtroom, the church, the town hall, the park, and the home.

Differences are not value judgments; they do not mean better or worse. To acknowledge difference is not to expose weakness but rather to celebrate uniqueness. Unique differences are the building blocks of philosophy and dreams, great art, poetry, and science: they are the essence of our God-created humanity.

Day 264

Blessings on the merciful! You'll receive mercy yourselves.
—Matthew 5:7

Brainy Tip: We are designed to love each other.

In so many ways, much of our interaction gets lost in translation, and we're left to piece together what just happened. In those moments, misunderstandings, unmet expectations, and unresolved issues come together to create toxic thoughts that, over time, poison relationships. With only a series of clues and undesirable outcomes, we're left to try to figure out what actually happened.

We're all different. We don't process things the same way. If we view and interpret our spouse's, colleague's, child's, or friend's actions on the basis of our own motivations and intentions, then we'll misunderstand, end up hurt, and likely lash out. But if we take a moment and reflect that what she said wasn't what we heard and what he thought wasn't what we assumed, then grace, forgiveness, and love can prevail.

God has wired you for love, not conflict. By listening to what science has to say and applying God's Word, you can reach soaring heights as you learn to understand your spouse, colleague, son, daughter, friend—and yourself.

Day 265

But mercy triumphs over judgment.—James 2:13

> **Brainy Tip:** The quality of our relationships is determined by the quality of our judgment of others.

Don't let the often puzzling and confusing tendencies of other people frustrate you. They are a mystery—but don't see them as a helplessly complicated, unsolvable puzzle. Instead, treat the mystery as an invitation to an exciting adventure—a journey of discovery that will lead you to a new place and change you along the way. We serve a magnificent Creator who loves us so much that he makes each of us unique.

Learning how to embrace our differences can be life changing, and it increases brain function and intelligence to boot! Every one of us has a wide variety of relationships, and all of these relationships require growth in order to be healthy. We're brothers, sisters, mothers, daughters, fathers, sons, coworkers, friends, neighbors, business partners, coaches, athletes, and on and on and on. As we invest in, grow, strengthen, and develop those relationships, the quality of our lives is transformed.

Day 266

So fasten your belts—the belts of your minds! Keep yourselves under control. Set your hope completely on the grace that will be given you when Jesus the Messiah is revealed. —1 Peter 1:13

Brainy Tip: Monitoring your thoughts is essential for your health.

Controlling your thoughts sounds great, but how do you do it? You start by looking at your mental processes. And no, you do not crack open your skull like an egg and have a look at what is going on inside your brain! It is possible, however, to learn about your mental processes through thinking about your thinking and choosing what to think about. This is not only possible, it's essential.

What does controlling our thinking look like? Evaluate whether your thoughts give you a sense of peace or make you worried. If a particular thought concerns you, think about something else every time that thought pops up. Thinking about something else allows you to reconceptualize the disturbing thought. This is essential for a healthy mind, body, and life.

Day 267

The aim of this is for you all to be like-minded, sympathetic and loving to one another, tender-hearted and humble.—1 Peter 3:8

Brainy Tip: The Holy Spirit can help us love each other.

But you don't know how hard it is to love that person! You do not know what they have done to me! If you find yourself thinking that, I understand. People can be difficult. Without God's wisdom and guidance, we are all left to love and understand the people in our lives from the reservoir of our own kindness and compassion. And for most of us, that well will never be deep enough. We can't love others the way God's called us to through our own strength and willpower—we need the strength, mercy, and love of the Holy Spirit to guide our thoughts and lead us.

Practice reaching out and loving people who are not always easy to love. Think of how amazing and how focused you feel when you make the effort to truly reach out to someone and try to understand that difficult person. The insights you gain into yourself may surprise you!

Day 268

It is in vain that you rise up early and go late to rest, eating the bread of anxious toil; for he gives sleep to his beloved.
—Psalm 127:2

Brainy Tip: Impossible expectations can impede our ability to think clearly and succeed.

Toxic thoughts and chaotic, haphazard thinking come in many guises. On the surface, a thought such as *I must do well* or *I must finish this in the next thirty minutes* seems all right, but when you look at it closely and analyze the feelings it generates, you will see how the thought may not be serving you well at the point you are at. Demanding unrealistic performance from yourself and others, for instance, puts your mind and body into toxic stress mode, which has a negative effect on your brain and body health. This type of pressure can also lead to haphazard, distracted thinking, which certainly doesn't help matters!

Day 269

That's how you must shine your light in front of people! Then they will see what wonderful things you do, and they'll give glory to your father in heaven. —Matthew 5:16

Brainy Tip: When you torment yourself with toxic thinking, you damage your brain.

How many could-have, would-have, or should-have statements have you uttered today? How many if-onlys? How many times have you replayed a bad conversation or situation in your head, thinking about how it could have gone differently? How many times have you worried about something you couldn't control? How much time do you spend speculating? Do thoughts just run uncontrollably through your brain? Are you honest with yourself or do you run from your thoughts and feelings? Do you just go through the motions, not really committed to a goal, saying one thing but meaning another? Is your thinking distorted? Have you formed a personal identity around a problem or disease you are facing? Do you speak about "my arthritis" or "my heart problem"? Do you ever make comments like "Nothing ever goes right for me" or "I always mess up"? Do you battle with remembering things? With learning?

If you answered yes to any one of these questions, you are human! We all face challenges, and we all need to learn how to consciously control our thought lives, every moment of every day. Mind-body research increasingly points to the fact that consciously controlling your thoughts is one of the best ways of detoxing your brain and your life, so stop tormenting yourself with all the "what ifs" of life.

Day 270

And this is what I'm praying: that your love may overflow still more and more, in knowledge and in all astute wisdom.
—Philippians 1:9

Brainy Tip: Improving your thinking improves your intelligence.

When you use your mind to consciously take control of your thought life, you will find that it does not take long for the benefits to show. Studies show that a positive thinking environment can lead to significant structural changes in the brain's cortex in just four days, and the changes don't stop there! Your brain continues to change in a positive direction as long as you keep moving forward in the right direction.

Frequent, positive, and challenging learning experiences can actually increase intelligence in a relatively short amount of time. My own research has demonstrated that learning potential can be increased 35 to 75 percent if people are taught how to understand the mind-brain and body connection and to deliberately think in ways that encourage learning and memory formation (see my book *Switch On Your Brain*). Detoxing the brain by controlling your thought life won't only make you feel better but will also make you smarter—and being smarter will help you choose to follow the way of God's love.

Day 271

We must run the race that lies in front of us, and we must run it patiently.—Hebrews 12:1

> **Brainy Tip:** Being patient does wonders for the structure of the brain.

We readily accept that it takes time to develop skill and expertise in a sport, yet when it comes to the mind, this wisdom often seems to disappear from our mental logic. We get stuck in an endless cycle of cram learning for an exam or for work and then forgetting the information the next day. Research on neuroplasticity, including mine, reveals that to develop new habits takes cycles of sixty-three days, minimum, not twenty-one days. Most people give up within the first five to seven days!

Real, long-term change that leads to transformed lives comes from persisting for at least three cycles of twenty-one days, or sixty-three days, since it takes two months for new cells to form. There is no shortcut when it comes to mind and brain change. Be patient!

Day 272

My yoke is easy to wear; my load is easy to bear.—Matthew 11:30

> **Brainy Tip:** As science progresses, researchers are getting glimpses into the minute, intricate structures of the brain that highlight its complex quantum nature. This quantum nature responds to our customized mode of thinking—our innate, intangible humanness.

God has given you everything you need to change—a yoke that is easy to bear with your customized, quantum nature.

Sometimes the idea of changing our thinking or the way we live our lives is frightening. Can we even do it? You may feel like you have been this way for such a long time that you cannot change, that God is just asking too much. But why would God tell us to do something if it weren't possible? He wouldn't. Because he's told us to do it, we can be sure that he's also given us the power not only to obey in one moment but to consistently live this way over time.

Day 273

Don't you know that when people run on the racetrack everybody runs, but only one person gets the prize? Run in such a way that you'll win it.—1 Corinthians 9:24

Brainy Tip: If you run a race expecting to win, you are more likely to win. Expectations can shape realities.

If we harness our natural ability to persevere, developing our iron will like athletes before a competition, we can use our minds—that is, our ability to think, feel, and choose—to achieve our goals and be successful in school, work, and life. If you *expect* that you will know the answers to a test because you have studied hard, for instance, you are more likely to study hard even if you don't feel like it, because your determination encourages you to keep on keeping on. As you move into an expectation mindset, you activate the neural wiring of the brain to succeed!

Day 274

Well then: I don't run in an aimless fashion! I don't box like someone punching the air! No: I give my body rough treatment, and make it my slave, in case, after announcing the message to others, I myself should end up being disqualified.—1 Corinthians 9:26–27

Brainy Tip: Willpower is essential to the life well lived.

Are you one of those people who sets ten alarms at three-minute intervals just to get up in the morning? How much willpower does it take to get out of your warm, cozy bed? A lot, I know! Often, we have to push ourselves to do something we don't feel like doing. We all have willpower, because we all have things we have to do that we don't want to do. Willpower is the mindset that allows us to persevere even if we do not feel like persevering.

We can use our willpower to change our *thoughts* about a physical or a mental act. These choices impact our brain and body, giving us the energy to pursue a task and achieve our goal.

Day 275

You'll bring in the harvest at the proper time, if you don't become weary.—Galatians 6:9

> **Brainy Tip:** We can resist the temptation to give up.

We all experience periods in our lives when our plans seem to dissolve into nothing, and the desire to give up sounds like a mythical siren's call, demanding that we abandon our hopes and dreams and dive into the deep. It is at times like these that we need to be on guard. We need to observe our thinking and catch ourselves when we feel like quitting!

When we feel like we are in a dark place and that we have nothing, we need to think of how powerful our minds are and choose to persevere. We must not allow toxic feelings to control us. We should only allow healthy feelings to rule over our thinking! We need to think of ways we can build up our willpower to do things we do not always feel like doing, particularly when we feel tired or like a failure.

What are your "plugs"? How can you motivate yourself to start, or finish, a task? Write down your ideas and put them into action when you feel like you cannot carry on. Remember, you are more than capable of succeeding at whatever you put your mind to.

Day 276

Through him [Jesus] we have been allowed to approach, by faith, into this grace in which we stand; and we celebrate the hope of the glory of God.—Romans 5:2

Brainy Tip: Faith can be good for your mental and physical health.

Faith is not a delusion. Choosing to have faith in God's promises, believing that the Holy Spirit will help you renew your mind, can help you persevere through hard times and enjoy the good times.

Our beliefs can actually help us live long and successful lives. In the "blue zones," regions in the world where there is the highest concentration of centenarians, spirituality is one of the key components associated with health and longevity![1] Belief in a higher power can foster a strong sense of community and hope, helping people feel that they are living for something greater than themselves—and greater than their problems or insecurities.

Of course, like everything in life, we can use spirituality in a negative sense, but the comfort and peace that come with being part of a spiritual community can be invaluable for our mental and physical wellbeing. Science, after all, does not hold a monopoly on truth. Our faith is another vantage point that allows us to seek God in *all* his glory.

Day 277

You heard that it was said, "Love your neighbor and hate your enemy." But I tell you: love your enemies! Pray for people who persecute you! That way, you'll be children of your father in heaven!—Matthew 5:43–45

Brainy Tip: Your brain and body function best as you develop a support mindset.

An essential component to having a support mindset is the power of healing in groups and reaching out to help others, as opposed to just getting help for yourself. High levels of social support predict longevity even more reliably than healthy eating and regular exercise do, while low levels of social support can be as damaging as high blood pressure.

For individuals facing difficulties in their lives (i.e., *everyone*), isolation can be lethal. Social support is crucial if we want to learn how to manage our emotions and deal with the vagaries of life. Indeed, strong, supportive relationships allow us to persevere through hard times.

Day 278

Keep yourselves in the love of God, as you wait for our Lord Jesus the Messiah to show you the mercy which leads to the life of the age to come.—Judah 21

Brainy Tip: Operating in love means that your words, actions, and body language match what you think about—that is, your intentions.

We don't just speak with our words. Our eyes, eyebrows, shoulders, back, arms, hands, legs, and feet can all talk. They can whisper and shout too. Half of all communication is non-verbal. That means how we say what we say is as important as what we actually say—maybe even more so.

Like the careless words we can speak if we fail to consider their impact, our nonverbal communication will tell the truth of what we believe deep down in our subconscious. That's why it's so important to get congruency between what we are thinking and what we are saying, because in the long run the truth will come out. It is so important to love authentically and unconditionally. No matter how sneaky you think you are, you can't hide your attitudes. No thought is harmless. Even when we're able to disguise what we really mean with our words, our eye-talk, body language, and gestures will tell the truth.

Day 279

And now, dear Lady, I ask you, not as though I were writing you a new commandment, but the one we had from the very beginning, that we should love one another. This is love: that we should behave in accordance with his commandments. And this is the commandment, just as you heard it from the very start, that we should behave in accordance with it. —2 John 5–6

> **Brainy Tip:** It is important that we think according to the love of the Messiah and not just say we love others.

When we are attentive, supportive, gentle, and encouraging with our body language, we can provide peace, understanding, and love without saying a single word. On the other hand, our posture and facial expressions can also be confrontational, aggressive, demeaning, or rude.

Many times our body language betrays our words—our mouths may be saying "I'm sorry, I didn't mean to upset you," while our bodies are saying, "What are you crying about? It's not that big of a deal." If we fail to understand the basics of nonverbal language, we'll continue to send mixed messages that will damage our relationships or at least keep them from getting stronger.

Day 280

*I wait for the LORD, my soul waits, and in his word I hope;
my soul waits for the Lord more than those who watch for
the morning, more than those who watch for the morning.*
—Psalm 130:5–6

Brainy Tip: What you anticipate can affect what comes to pass.

Your insula, working with the rest of the brain, responds
to your anticipating what something will feel like before it
happens. For example, on a cold day, your insula gets your
body ready by pumping blood to where it will be needed and
adjusting your metabolism. This happens on a psychological
level as well, as you anticipate the emotional content of how
you feel now and how you may feel in a particular situation.

Your insula is particularly active when you build a connection in your mind between the existing memory (thought) of
a circumstance or event and what is about to happen—that
is, as you predict and anticipate. This can be a good or a bad
thing. It is good if the thought network the anticipation is
based on is healthy, but not so good if it's toxic. In the latter
case, the toxic anticipation and prediction can allow your
fears to get the better of you, causing a negative reaction in
your brain and body.

Your anticipations can lead to realities!

Day 281

The mind of the righteous ponders how to answer, but the mouth of the wicked pours out evil.—Proverbs 15:28

Brainy Tip: "Thinker" moments are good for our mental health!

The average person spends up to eight hours a day using technology. Some of the worst effects of electronic devices seem to be mitigated when devices are used less than two hours a day. Find ways to limit your use of technology throughout the day, and increase your "thinker" moments!

Thinker moments teach you how to live the examined, love-filled life. As your mind wanders, think about what you are thinking and your own experiences, perhaps writing about your thoughts in a journal or on a notepad. Evaluate whether your thoughts give you a sense of peace or make you worried. If your thoughts concern you, think differently about the same thing, every time that thought or those thoughts pop up. In other words, reconceptualize the disturbing thought or thoughts.

These moments develop your intelligence, increase your health, give you a sense of peace, and help you use your mind and brain efficiently. So when you don't feel like being a "thinker," remember that these moments make you smarter and better equipped to handle life!

Day 282

No creature remains hidden before God. All are naked, laid bare before the eyes of the one to whom we must present an account.—Hebrews 4:13

Brainy Tip: The sooner you deal with negative, toxic thoughts, the sooner you remove their power over your life.

I want to renew my mind, you may be thinking, *but where do I begin? How do I even start trying to sort out my mental life? How do I change my thoughts?*

Because of the design of the brain, you can reconceptualize (redesign) thoughts that are holding you back by deciding what thought you would rather have. You then work toward eliminating the toxic thought and building something better. Start with acknowledging and articulating the thoughts that are weighing you down—ones that don't serve any useful purpose beyond keeping you stuck in a rut. Now ask yourself questions rather than issuing commands to yourself—this is a much more effective way to reconceptualize, because it opens up exploration and creative possibility and distances you from what you are thinking, giving you a safe space for change. You can also label your emotions in a nonjudgmental way to give yourself some distance from them in order to deal with them.

Remember, you cannot hide your thoughts! Sooner or later, what you are thinking, choosing, and feeling will come to the surface. The sooner you deal with negative, toxic thoughts, the sooner you remove their power over your life.

Day 283

"You shall love your neighbor as yourself." No other commandment is greater than these.—Mark 12:31

Brainy Tip: Watch what you say when you are alone.

Become intentionally mindful about what you say, not only when you are with other people but also when you are by yourself. When you do this, the internal networks of your brain fire up and your inner peace and mental health will grow. Start replacing negative statements with positive ones, thinking about the kind of change you want to see in your life.

You might want to reconceptualize your self-talk. Remind yourself that you are a work in progress and that's totally fine. Point yourself in the direction of achievable growth—what is realistic for you? What can you do with where you are in life? Perhaps tell yourself something like, "Every moment I'm making an effort to be more conscious about how I manage my time."

Acknowledge the fact that you are evolving and that you can choose to create a better future for yourself. It is important to remember that you cannot love others or truly show them grace if you do not love yourself or show yourself grace.

293

Day 284

After all, the spirit given to us by God isn't a fearful spirit;
it's a spirit of power, love, and prudence.—2 Timothy 1:7

Brainy Tip: You cannot hide what you are feeling, but you can control what you are feeling.

The first vital step in controlling your emotions is recognizing *you have control* over your emotions! You build them into your brain with your mind. Emotions are not universal or preprogrammed but rather unique to you. They don't happen to you; emotions are made *by you*.

You do not have to wear your heart on your sleeve or let everything hang out. You do, however, have to be honest with yourself. This is an evolving process of working out what you are feeling and how to deal with these emotions.

You need to express emotions appropriately, in an environment that is safe, accepting, and nonjudgmental. I suggest you create lists of "safe," "less safe," and "not safe" people. The first group is people you know you can trust (loved ones, a really close friend, a counselor). The second group is people with whom you feel you can share to an extent, but not everything. The third group is people you definitely won't talk to because you know it will backfire.

Day 285

Rather, celebrate! You are sharing the sufferings of the Messiah. Then, when his glory is revealed, you will celebrate with real, exuberant joy.—1 Peter 4:13

Brainy Tip: Enjoying the journey enables you to truly enjoy the destination.

Choose to be happy, pushing through a challenge and enjoying the process of developing your understanding and abilities. If you fail, pick yourself up, even if you don't feel like it! Despite how you initially feel, choosing to be happy will become the energy source that keeps you going. Think of having your own personal happiness meter—check it as often as you need to. If it's dropping, stop, breathe, and ask yourself why. Then choose to overcome whatever you are facing—choose to change it.

Don't allow yourself to think *I will be so happy when this is over.* Learn to enjoy the start, the middle, and the end! Of course, it's okay to experience different emotions moving toward peaceful acceptance—if you are happy all the time, you do not grow in understanding. Our struggles have a way of teaching us to be truly happy in the long run by showing us what true happiness is.

Day 286

We know, in fact, that God works all things together for good to those who love him, who are called according to his purpose.—Romans 8:28

Brainy Tip: Don't let your failures define you.

Think of failure as knowledge obtained, even if it is knowledge of what not to do! Never label something a complete failure. Everything is a teaching moment, developing your mind and your character.

Don't let the time it takes for the attainment of a skill, for a change of mindset, to learn to control emotions, or to forgive discourage you from keeping on. If things take longer than you planned, adjust—don't panic. If you panic, you may end up undoing what you have just done and putting your brain and body into toxic stress! Take life one day at a time, breathe, and have faith in the incredible mind God has given you.

Day 287

For this reason, since we have this work entrusted to us in accordance with the mercy we have received, we don't lose heart.—2 Corinthians 4:1

> **Brainy Tip:** When you fall, pick yourself up. If you focus on your failures, you will continue to fail.

We live in a world of probabilities. We have the creative power in our mind to transform these possibilities into realities. *Choose* to develop a mindset that allows you to perceive possibilities, so that the wired-for-love design of your brain can be activated to respond.

Stop yourself immediately if you catch yourself thinking *There is no way out* or *I am a failure*. Take that thought captive! Replace it with *I cannot be a failure because I am wired for success. I am designed to reflect God's glory into the world*. Do not let what other people have said about you, or what you have said about yourself, hold you back from living out God's plan for your life.

Day 288

See, I am the LORD, the God of all flesh; is anything too hard for me?—Jeremiah 32:27

Brainy Tip: You can choose to see possibilities where other people see failures.

Do you spend more time counting your blessings or more time focusing on what is missing from your life? Do you find yourself saying things like "I didn't manage to see that or do that" instead of "I did manage to see this and do that"?

Think about what you say before you say it, and if you have already started saying something negative, watch what you say and catch those thoughts, change them, and say something positive before you start complaining and damaging your brain, body, and relationships! *Choose* to see the glass as half full, not half empty. You have the power of God inside you!

Day 289

Just as each of you has received a gift, so you should use it for ministry one to another, as good stewards of God's many-sided grace.—1 Peter 4:10

> **Brainy Tip:** You are an important member of your community. You can do something no one else can do.

Community and social integration are essential to mental and physical health, especially when you find yourself in a dark place or feel that you are a failure. When you feel burdened with work or emotionally challenged, or are going through something, try stopping for a moment and helping someone else, even if it is just to listen, hug, or encourage them. Send an email or text to someone telling them you are thinking of them, or invite someone to dinner instead of eating alone.

Choose to wake up every morning and ask yourself, *Who can I help today?* Think about what you could do to get out of the house and foster community in your area. Perhaps start a book club or arrange dinner parties and invite someone new each time. Get to know your neighbors and invite them for a walk or for coffee, or join a local community or spiritual center. The possibilities are endless!

You don't have to save the world. You need to start simply with purpose, and this can be as simple as looking outside your front door into your neighborhood, grocery store, gym, or church. If you are fulfilled on a personal level, you will touch someone else, and this will spiral into a world effect. You matter, and what you think matters!

Day 290

Cast your burden on the LORD, and he will sustain you; he will never permit the righteous to be moved.—Psalm 55:22

Brainy Tip: Change the way you think about stress.

Stress is something that can enhance, rather than diminish, your performance. Each time you feel yourself teetering on the brink of toxic stress, visualize those blood vessels around your heart dilating and pumping blood and oxygen into your brain. Visualize neurotransmitters being released, and see it all working together to help you focus and think with clarity to react in the best way. To help you get perspective, speak with your friends or family (even if it is just a phone call or a text message).

In fact, when you face a challenge, tell yourself how good stress can be for you! Think of all the positive benefits (mentioned above) that good stress can have on your body. Tell yourself that you will have more clarity for thought if you make stress work for you. Perhaps write down the benefits of a healthy reaction to stress and keep it on you, reading it when you feel challenged. See stress as something that enhances, rather than diminishes, your performance. Remember, you have an incredibly powerful mind!

Day 291

Let us, as well, stir up one another's minds to energetic effort in love and good works . . . we must encourage one another, and all the more as you can see the great day coming closer.
—Hebrews 10:24–25

Brainy Tip: We all think differently. These differences are complementary.

We have all experienced moments when our thinking gets the better of us. Perhaps we are alone at home or cannot sleep, and suddenly our mind bombards us with every wrong we have done and every mistake we have made. It is in moments like these that community becomes essential to our wellbeing.

Thinking is a process and goes through a cycle, just like digestion. In the same way that food is *digested* and the nutritional content is *used* by our cells for life to take place, information has to be digested through thinking before it can be used in a "nutritionally" meaningful way, forming memory. Information that comes in through our senses is digested through our customized way of thinking. My way of thinking is different from yours—not better, just different. *Completeness* actually comes in these differences. Say, for example, we are having a bad day. Often, asking a friend for advice or a loved one for their perspective can change the way we feel and help us see our situation in a different, brighter light.

Our unique way of thinking brings us together and helps us serve each other and the God who created all of us. We are better, and stronger, together!

Day 292

It is the one spirit, the same one, whose work produces all these things, and the spirit gives different gifts to each one in accordance with the spirit's own wishes.—1 Corinthians 12:11

Brainy Tip: We each have our own customized way of thinking.

No two individuals are alike. Studies of twins, for example, show us that even though they have identical DNA, they are different because they think differently. Their customized mode of thinking, which results in a distinct way of building memory and therefore learning, changes their genetic expression, thereby changing what they say and do. Twins, even if they are identical, can have incredibly different likes and dislikes, behavior, and life choices. They even have different susceptibility to disease.

We are not merely our genes or our biology. Our thoughts make us who we are. What do your thoughts say about you?

Day 293

For where there is jealousy and contention, there you will get unruly behavior and every kind of evil practice.—James 3:16

Brainy Tip: You are designed to be you.

If you don't operate in your unique way of thinking, you will work against who you are at your core. If you try to be like someone else, your mental and physical health will be compromised, because your thoughts can affect the way your genes are expressed. You can experience frustration, losing your clarity of thought and direction. You can lose your sense of inner peace, which in turn affects your sense of achievement. Your ability to communicate, learn, and function at school, at work, and in life will be negatively impacted. You cannot truly be anyone but yourself.

Day 294

Love is kind, knows no jealousy, makes no fuss, is not puffed up.—1 Corinthians 13:4

Brainy Tip: When you rejoice in who you are, you can truly love others.

As you think in your customized mode of thinking, you can literally repair your brain and body, because the neuroplastic nature of your brain is resetting to its default mode.

Every cell in your body contains your full makeup of DNA. Your unique thinking can actually switch genes on, influencing how the DNA functions. The effective functioning of your genes is largely dependent on the effective functioning of your thinking, which kicks in when you learn how to use your customized way of thinking.

You would make a lousy someone else, but you make a great you when you operate in your customized thinking! You need to realize that you are wonderful just the way you are. You need to recognize the genius in yourself and the genius in others.

Day 295

[Love] doesn't force its rightful claim, doesn't rage or bear a grudge, doesn't cheer at others' harm, rejoices, rather, in the truth.—1 Corinthians 13:5–6

Brainy Tip: We damage our brain when we communicate in an unkind way.

In today's world, it often seems we do not know how to talk to each other. We all have different opinions; we all think differently; we all speak and act differently. Indeed, one of the greatest challenges can be interacting with people because they do not think like us! We can misunderstand what another person is trying to communicate to us, and vice versa. This misunderstanding often leads to arguments, or worse.

When we understand how we think, however, we can recognize that others think, feel, and choose differently as well. We recognize that these differences are not inherently bad but rather wonderfully good! We learn not to feel threatened by people who do not think, act, or speak like us. Turn this around and see it as enhancing your own genius—and this is exactly what research in mind and brain science is showing us! We will become more understanding, allowing us to develop and maintain a strong sense of community, which is critical to human happiness and success. As social animals, we cannot function well if we cannot communicate, and we cannot love well if we cannot communicate well.

Day 296

Much will be required from one who is given much; if some-one is entrusted with much, even more will be expected in return.—Luke 12:48

Brainy Tip: We are responsible for our choices.

Your amygdala *didn't* make you do it. Wait, do what? You are not your brain structures. Your amygdala—or any other part of your brain—cannot make you say or do anything. Parts of your brain do not control you; they are simply structures within the brain with specific neurophysiological functions that become more or less active *in response to* you expressing what it feels like inside. They are activated by your perception, your unique mode of thinking. The brain is like a complex quantum computer that *reflects and expresses* the mind (or inner life) of a human being.

We are made in the image of the Creator, yet we are often surprised that we have the power and responsibility to cre-ate. We cause structural changes in our brains through the way we think, feel, and choose. Through our customized way of thinking, we create matter with our minds. We need to take this power seriously. We can bring heaven or hell to earth—the choice is ours.

Day 297

God is the God, not of chaos, but of peace.
—1 Corinthians 14:33

> **Brainy Tip:** Through our choices we can develop our peace and understanding.

Our thought life is a "stream of consciousness" with thousands of individual thoughts blending together. We can control what we allow into our heads. We are able to evaluate the individual frames of thought by self-regulating the stream of consciousness. When we get distracted by external influences and toxic reactions to life, however, our ability to self-regulate can get affected, with negative consequences for our mental and physical health.

When we learn to understand and control how we think, we are *retraining* our self-regulatory function, which allows us to monitor our thinking in the long term. No matter how chaotic your mind is, you can control your thinking!

Day 298

Well then, we have gifts that differ in accordance with the grace that has been given to us, and we must use them appropriately. —Romans 12:6

Brainy Tip: We all think, speak, and act in different ways. We all have a unique perception of the world.

Our views of the world are reflected in the architecture of our brains because we built them into the brain with our thoughts. We all do this, but with different results because we are all different. From the macro level of the structure of each part of the brain, to the micro level of the neurons, to the subatomic level, to the quantum level of vibrations, we are all unique. The basic genome is nearly the same in all of us, but it is utilized differently across the body and among individuals. Even our proteins vibrate in different ways!

If we *mindfully* tune in to our ability to think, feel, and choose—that is, our customized thinking—and choose to pay attention to our thoughts, we can understand how we think, the very core of who we are! Our customized way of thinking pervades all our choices, and it's a powerful uniqueness that we each need to harness and use to our advantage.

Day 299

No discipline seems to bring joy at the time, but only sorrow. Later, though, it produces fruit, the peaceful fruit of righteousness, for those who are trained by it.—Hebrews 12:11

Brainy Tip: Discipline and diligence are essential for mind renewal.

We need to take responsibility for thinking to succeed in life. No one is going to do it for us. Discipline is not always easy, and there are days when we will feel like giving up when we feel any degree of "sorrow." A lot of people tend to give up a difficult task after just a few days! But our minds are designed to persevere. In fact, perseverance and diligence are the only ways to achieve new skill levels and grow your intelligence. Success is not momentary; success, the "fruit" of our labors, is the result of a lifestyle of growth and development.

Day 300

Show me your treasure, and I'll show you where your heart is.—Matthew 6:21

> **Brainy Tip:** What you focus on the most, what you love, will direct your thinking.

Every moment of every day we are merging with our environment. Through thinking, feeling, and choosing, we are learning and planting thoughts, which are real, physical things, into the brain. This happens in our minds 24/7; when we are asleep, our brain sorts out the thoughts we built during the day (a type of mental housekeeping). We are incredibly intellectual beings, even when we are not aware of what is going on in our minds.

It is therefore so important that we recognize the power our environment has over us—if we give it this power. If we go about our lives in a haphazard and reactive way, we run the risk of allowing external influences to run through our minds unimpeded. These influences have the potential to shape the way we view and interact with the world. We need to recognize that the fact the brain can change also means that if we are not directing this change through our thinking, something else will be.

Day 301

An intelligent mind acquires knowledge, and the ear of the wise seeks knowledge.—Proverbs 18:15

> **Brainy Tip:** Learning creates and redesigns memory.

Learning is the creative reconceptualization of knowledge. It is the creation and redesigning of memory. It is controlled by active and dynamic self-regulation—deep, intentional thought. It has the quality of personal involvement, it is pervasive, and its essence is meaning and purpose. What we learn determines the meaning of our lives, since it shapes our worldview, which is the mindset filter through which we see everything.

Remember, whatever we focus on the most will grow and influence our perspectives and belief systems (or worldviews). As the saying goes, we become what we love. This can be both a positive and a negative experience.

What are you learning? What gives your life meaning and purpose? What knowledge are you seeking? What influences the way you understand and interact with the world? Do you have a "heaven-to-earth" mindset?

Day 302

If we confess our sins, he is faithful and just, and will forgive us our sins, and cleanse us from all unrighteousness. If we say that we have not sinned, we make him out to be a liar, and his word is not in us.—1 John 1:9–10

Brainy Tip: We cannot change until we admit that we need to change.

We can change nothing until we fully comprehend what needs to be changed—where we have missed the mark and lost our way. Just as every action first begins with a thought, we, as the children of the Creator of this beautiful universe, have to renew our own minds before we can restore and renew the world for God's kingdom.

We have to admit that there are problems we have to face before we can beat them, quit the broken system, and change our world for the better. Pretending we do not have problems, or trying to sweep issues under the carpet, will not help anyone, especially ourselves. Change starts when we take a good look in the mirror.

Day 303

Or don't you know that your body is a temple of the holy spirit within you, the spirit God gave you, so that you don't belong to yourselves? You were quite an expensive purchase! So glorify God in your body.—1 Corinthians 6:19–20

Brainy Tip: If we want a healthy life, we need to have a healthy mind.

If we do not have a healthy mind, then nothing else in our life will be healthy, no matter how many squats we do, how many Bible verses we know, how many hours we sleep, or how many kale salads we eat. True, lasting health incorporates the elements of choice and its consequences, bringing all thoughts into captivity to the Messiah, renewing the mind, being led by the Holy Spirit, respecting the temple God has given us, and respecting the earth God has entrusted to us. It is about taking responsibility for the power we have in our minds, the power to create, and using this power to reflect his glory and bring life into a hurting world.

Day 304

The LORD will guide you continually, and satisfy your needs in parched places, and make your bones strong; and you shall be like a watered garden, like a spring of water, whose waters never fail.—Isaiah 58:11

Brainy Tip: True happiness comes from internal satisfaction.

As a culture, we have become so accustomed to our current, global system of "more, more, more" and "now, now, now" that it has become a part of our nonconscious minds. When was the last time you thought about where your food came from? Or who made your clothes? Or if you really need the latest smartphone and why? Or what exactly you are working for? Or why you chose your job? Or if you feel spiritually fulfilled? Or why you are dating that person? How often do you stop to smell the roses and think about the beauty you see in a single flower? When was the last time you felt satisfied with where you are in life and with what you have?

Happiness is not measured by how many things you have or how fabulous your life looks on social media but by how satisfied you are with your life and where your life is headed, even when times are challenging. This kind of satisfaction, which cannot be bought at the store or online, is the foundation of your mental and physical wellbeing—it is based in God's love and it will never fail. It will give you the strength to keep on keeping on!

Day 305

You'll be able to tell them by the fruit they bear: you don't find grapes growing on thorn-bushes, do you, or figs on thistles? Well, in the same way, good trees produce good fruit, and bad trees produce bad fruit. Actually, good trees can't produce bad fruit, nor can bad ones produce good fruit!
—Matthew 7:16–19

Brainy Tip: True change can be seen in the fruit of your life.

We need to take personal responsibility for our lifestyles. Of course, we all make mistakes, and we can rest assured knowing that God, in his gracious and loving way, has built backup systems into our brains and bodies that will pull us out of potential danger and heal us. After all, stressing about making mistakes is toxic to our mental and physical health! But if we knowingly continue down a path of choosing toxic, negative thinking patterns, we should not be surprised when the consequences are far from what we desire.

Yes, God forgives us, but we have to repent, which essentially means to change our mind, which in turn changes our behavior. We cannot treat the Creator of the universe as a "get out of jail free" card or a bottled genie ready for our wish. Remember: what we think, we are.

Day 306

The warfare we're engaged in, you see, isn't against flesh and blood. It's against the leaders, against the authorities, against the powers that rule the world in this dark age, against the wicked spiritual elements in the heavenly places.
—Ephesians 6:12

> **Brainy Tip:** We can never let down our guard when it comes to our thinking.

It is foolhardy to believe that we can live our lives however we choose and, when problems arise, just sit back and ask God why this is happening to us and tell everyone we are under spiritual attack. We are always under attack on every front. St. Paul says we are *in* a war, not going to war. It is a war to win over our minds and our lives. We are part of this battle of restoration; we are called to be God's heirs, soldiers, and high priests, extending his love and forgiveness in the world. This is what it means to be true followers of the Messiah, who extended God's love and mercy into the world by conquering sin and death. We are called to bring heaven to earth, and this does not happen without a struggle, mentally and physically.

Day 307

So, then, if anyone knows the right thing to do, but doesn't do it, it becomes sin for them.—James 4:17

Brainy Tip: With knowledge comes responsibility.

I think a frightening mentality among many people today is a pervasive view of the world as fallen and hopeless, despite the fact that the Messiah has already made all things new. We have the God-given responsibility to care for the earth—the whole world is waiting for the followers of Jesus to fully appropriate their identity as God's heirs and take responsibility for creation.

The world is being restored—a restoration that began with Jesus and will be completed with Jesus, and through us as his heirs. We were not created to stand by, complaining about the evil things we witness or hear about and exclaiming that we cannot wait to go to heaven and leave this wretched earth behind. We are supposed to bring heaven to earth, to apply God's love to the terrible things that make us want to hide our heads in the sand like spiritual ostriches. Yet once we know, we have a responsibility to act. As followers of the Messiah, we cannot say that it is impossible to escape or change the way things are, because we are called to change the way things are!

Day 308

Therefore, there is no condemnation for those in the Messiah, Jesus!—Romans 8:1

Brainy Tip: Uncontrolled guilt is toxic to the brain and body.

Sometimes, when we think of our thinking, we can get caught up in a negative spiral of guilt and condemnation. You must not let these feelings run through your mind unchecked! Uncontrolled guilt can put your body in toxic stress, negatively impacting your mental and physical health.

Indeed, guilt is destructive to the mind and brain and needs to be overridden, or it will keep you stuck in a rut of condemnation. It is a good idea to find the source of the guilt, because sometimes it is not a valid source—you may have been believing a lie!

Remember, we all need to observe and change the way we think on a daily basis—we all need to renew our minds. And when we think about the impact of our lifestyle choices, we improve the quality of our lifestyles, which will have a profound influence on the health of our spirits, minds, and bodies.

Day 309

Train children in the right way, and when old, they will not stray.—Proverbs 22:6

> **Brainy Tip:** Our children will follow our example.

Children will do what we do, not what we say. A parent's toxic lifestyle can predispose a child to a toxic lifestyle. Nourishing lifestyle patterns that foster healthy responses to life should be established at a young age. We especially need to teach our children about the power that is in their minds and how to handle it, even when it is difficult and time-consuming for everyone involved. Confused emotions and thoughts create disorders in the mind, which in turn will produce behaviors that are equally confused and self-destructive.

Create an environment that is open, safe, and nonjudgmental. Always be willing to listen to your children, and maybe even change the way you think, speak, and act. Just because you are the parent it does not mean you know everything.

Day 310

Create in me a clean heart, O God, and put a new and right spirit within me.—Psalm 51:10

Brainy Tip: The mind is more powerful than the brain.

Change in life-damaging patterns of behavior comes with choosing to change based on an awareness of the fundamental need to change. You are not a victim of what you think, say, and do, because you control what you think, say, and do.

The concept of a brain disease is very limiting and almost always gives a sense of hopelessness. It is the reductionistic view, one that says you are what your brain does and there is really nothing you alone can do about it. This is based on old, incorrect scientific research and a materialist philosophy that is antithetical to what the Bible and recent scientific research indicate.

A thinking disorder, on the other hand, brings hope in the sense that although there have been significant biological changes in the brain, the brain can change (neuroplasticity). The mind is more powerful than the brain: it directs change.

Day 311

I came so that they could have life—yes, and have it full to overflowing.—John 10:10

> **Brainy Tip:** It is never too late to change the way you think, speak, and act.

Choosing to change and quit a toxic thinking pattern can result in brain regrowth. A number of researchers have found that adult brain volume, which can be reduced by thinking disorders (or bad thinking habits), can also be regained through changing thinking patterns or mindsets. By choosing to change the way you think, you can literally regain gray matter in the brain!

When God said his plans for you are full of hope, he truly meant it. He really wants you to live the best life you can live. His love, mercy, and grace are never-ending. Regrow your brain in the right wired-for-love way!

Day 312

After you have suffered a little while, the God of all grace, who called you in the Messiah Jesus to the glory of his new age, will himself put you in good order, and will establish and strengthen you and set you on firm foundations.—1 Peter 5:10

> **Brainy Tip:** It takes time to wire a habit into the brain; it takes time to wire a habit out of the brain.

The signals that change our brains can be good or bad. The same plasticity (change in the brain) principles are employed as we wire in a good or a bad habit—this is called the plastic paradox.

Yet if the mind can change the brain, why do unhealthy thinking, speaking, and acting habits seem so hard to break? We used plasticity to build these habits over time; we used plasticity to implant them in our minds. As you well know, whatever you think about the most grows. Thus, by the same token, the same kind of effort goes into breaking the habit, but because we are reversing the tide, there is more effort involved.

Plasticity does not equal effortlessness. It is extremely hard work, but *anything worthwhile is hard work*. Plasticity means change, and true, lasting change is never effortless. Good, healthy signals equal good, healthy brain changes. Likewise, bad, unhealthy signals equal bad, unhealthy brain changes.

Day 313

*I am going to bring it recovery and healing; I will heal them
and reveal to them abundance of prosperity and security.*
—Jeremiah 33:6

Brainy Tip: Addiction means to be consumed by something.

We are designed to be consumed by love. Research shows
love is the top addiction, and more people die from loneliness and the lack of love than any other disease. Our brains
are wired to latch on to something, and that something is
God's "loveness." Any toxic addiction, whether it be to food,
drugs, or even a person, is the result of misplaced choice, or
disordered love.

Addiction is not a chronic, lifelong disease, as the current
biomedical model depicts it to be. Addiction to the wrong
thing happens when our natural addiction to love is thwarted
in some way. There is extensive evidence, particularly in popu-
lation studies, that the vast majority of people who quit toxic
addictions do so on their own through the *choice to change*
their thinking and harnessing their willpower.

Of course, God did not say that life would be easy and
carefree—it can never be when free will is involved. But Jesus
did come to set us free and give us life abundantly. He came to
heal us. God has made all things new in the Messiah. Jesus has
already won the victory. We were never created to just "cope."

Day 314

Rather, in every area of life let God know what you want, as you pray and make requests, and give thanks as well. And God's peace, which is greater than we can ever understand, will keep guard over your hearts and minds in King Jesus.
—Philippians 4:6–7

> **Brainy Tip:** We can overcome toxic addictions by changing the way we think.

When we focus on something or someone for long periods of time (worship or love it), the reward circuits in the brain become hijacked by our choices (mind), which change the brain physically. We can become addicted to anything if we pay it attention over a significant amount of time.

Wired-for-love reward circuits become distorted by negative thoughts and wrong lifestyle choices (and other environmental factors) in a circular feedback loop, and can certainly affect the clarity of the mind and our ability to tap into our full potential. Yet the mind is still stronger than the brain: Jesus said he would never give us any more than we are able to bear, and he has provided a way for us to bear it. The brain will rewire, or renew, in the direction the mind sends it. Hence the vast majority of people can and do quit addictions on a daily basis. Choosing to get out of a toxic addiction is what testimonies, and indeed miracles, are made of.

Day 315

He has sent me to announce release to the prisoners and sight to the blind, to set the wounded victims free, to announce the year of God's special favor.—Luke 4:18–19

Brainy Tip: We see in quantum physics that God has created a probabilistic, open-ended universe that allows us to free ourselves from negative thinking patterns.

There is an infinite set of possibilities of perception. Although this may sound complicated, it is essentially another way of describing free will and the power God has given us. We can choose life or death, blessings or curses.

Quantum physics is a mathematically based description of the open-mindedness of choice. Einstein once said that God does not play dice with the universe.[1] He was a classical physicist and believed in a rational universe with specific laws that determined everything that would happen. Einstein did not like the concept of an open universe and free will, which he called an illusion. However, according to quantum physics, it looks very much as though God does play dice, but in a loving and generous sense. He does not force us to love and serve him. He designed us as intelligent, unique reflections of his glorious image, free to choose how we want to live our lives. He took a risk giving us free will, but love inherently involves risks.

God came to set us free, not lock us in. We have to choose in this probabilistic, open-ended universe to be freed from negative thinking patterns; we play a role in our own freedom!

Day 316

You are all one in the Messiah, Jesus.—Galatians 3:28

Brainy Tip: There is an inseparable quantum connectedness of every part with every other part.

The creative freedom we have when we operate in love is a powerful reality, not an illusion. With our Perfect You we build thoughts that become realities. These realities are tremendously important, because everything is connected, first in God and then in each other. No matter how far apart in distance and time, all particles in a relationship affect each other; these relationships exist beyond space and time.

Every thought we think affects everyone else, and vice versa. Because everything was created in and through God, creation is entangled. And, as image-bearers, we have a particular effect on the world and each other. We all have a piece of God's eternity in us, and collectively we represent his eternal creation. He is the whole system and we are the parts in him. Like cells in the human body, we originate from one source but have different functions depending on who and where we are within a larger community.

Day 317

And [he] gave them authority over unclean spirits, to cast them out and to heal every disease and every sickness.
—Matthew 10:1

Brainy Tip: You have power over your life.

Remember, your mind controls your brain and your brain controls your body. If you want a healthy body, you need a healthy mind. Your intentional thinking, feeling, and choosing affects how the matter in your body behaves. Regardless of the way you have chosen to react in the past, painful toxic thoughts can be reconstructed, even toxic feelings you have been nursing for so long and are so familiar with you think they are normal. You can analyze them and rewire them because of the brain's neuroplasticity. You can heal yourself!

However, if you are not selectively paying attention to what you are thinking about in any given situation, you will become reactive and driven by whatever thoughts (and their dynamic emotional energy) come into your mind. Don't live in an impulsive, reactive way. Do not allow your life to control you when you have the power to control your life. Don't ignore the authority God has given you.

The apostle Paul wrote that we have to bring all thoughts into captivity unto Jesus. All means *all*. Never let any thought go unchecked through your mind.

Day 318

Wise warriors are mightier than strong ones, and those who have knowledge than those who have strength.
—Proverbs 24:5

Brainy Tip: Never stop asking questions.

Deep critical thinking, which I have researched for years, involves asking, answering, and discussing incoming sensory information and existing internal thoughts as they move into the conscious mind. This means we consider all the options from as detached and informed a position as possible. This is what it means to think objectively, or in quantum physics terms, get into superposition. Superposition involves stopping, standing back, observing our own thoughts and the information coming in through the five senses, setting up a dialogue with the Holy Spirit, considering all the options, and then choosing which thoughts we want to implant in our nonconscious minds.

If there is one piece of advice I can give anyone, it is that you should think carefully and deliberately about all the information you encounter and ask a lot of questions! Never let anyone tell you that you have no right to use your brain. Indeed, to ignore the power that is in your mind would be a great loss—to you and to the world!

Day 319

*Seek the L*ORD *and his strength, seek his presence continually.*—1 Chronicles 16:11

> **Brainy Tip:** Research on the regulatory aspect of the human genome, the 97 percent of who we are, hints at the power of the thought life to cause changes in our brains and bodies.

More than 97 percent of our genome is fulfilling vital functions in a regulatory manner. It specifically controls the switching on and off of genes. It is a language, operating like a genetic switch that controls the other 3 percent. Our DNA is essentially designed to react to the language of our thoughts and resultant words as well as the biological signals.

We are made in the image of a powerful God who brought the earth into existence with his words, and we have this power of words and language invested in us. The first task given to humanity was to name the animals, after all!

As we seek after the Lord, we strengthen our ability to direct the regulatory part of our genome correctly, because we learn to build the correct love language into our brains and bodies down to the level of our DNA.

Day 320

Brainy Tip: Light is a nonphysical wave made up of packets of energy called quanta, also known as photons.

Light is the energy, God's energy, in our DNA that has been present since the beginning of creation. Since God created space and time, he is beyond space and time, so everything we need as humans has been and is and will be provided for us. We, through the power of our God-given intellect, access what God has provided for us through the choices we make as we use our Perfect You.

In both science and life, God inspires us, and we laboriously investigate and explore the correct mix of the ingredients that allow us to uniquely reflect his glorious ideas. For example, God through the Holy Spirit will release a divine inspiration, a spiritual prompt, in someone to begin a process of exploration. This leads to the discovery of how the things of nature and man—God's creation—work.

God's creation is a literal "global informational structure" that represents tendencies for real wired-for-love events to occur, and in which the choice of which potentiality will be actualized in various places is in the hands of human agents. This is called a "quantum state of the universe." We are the light of the world, so use this light wisely!

Day 321

Bear with one another in love; be humble, meek, and patient in every way with one another. Make every effort to guard the unity that the spirit gives, with your lives bound together in peace.—Ephesians 4:2–3

Brainy Tip: If we want to change our relationships we need to change our thinking.

Often in a relationship, when two people have reacted in certain ways and have built toxic thoughts, all new communication is viewed through the filter of the previous painful interactions, and every future conversation is shaped by the experience of the previous encounter. That's why we need to deal with these toxic patterns in our relationships so we can truly be a community that fosters healthy, life-giving relationships, whether we are talking about a spouse, a friend, or merely a colleague at school or work.

If we do not change our thinking, we cannot change our relationships. But when we work together as God intended, we gain the benefit of the full range of his wisdom and insight, which allows us to enjoy the party, and life in general, to the fullest.

Day 322

Let me tell you this: on judgment day people will have to own up to every trivial word they say.—Matthew 12:36

Brainy Tip: Our words have power to injure people, mentally and physically.

"Sticks and stones may break my bones, but words can never hurt me." You and I both know this is not true. In many cases the painful impact of a word cuts deeper and lasts longer than the blow of a stick or a stone. I'm sure you've experienced emotional pain—it can be just as real as physical pain. But while most people realize the reality of emotional pain, most people don't understand how closely connected physical and emotional pain actually are.

The physical and emotional experience of pain is processed through the whole brain. Specifically, the insula, the anterior central gyrus, and the somatosensory cortex in the frontal lobe areas light up with both physical *and* emotional pain. In the brain, words and stones have the same impact! So watch not only how you act toward other people but also what you say! Your words have a real, physical effect in their brains.

Day 323

Do you see someone who is hasty in speech? There is more hope for a fool than for anyone like that.—Proverbs 29:20

Brainy Tip: Watch your words, for they reflect how you view God's precious creation.

Although we cannot be sure of the words that will be spoken over us in the future, we can choose whether or not to accept them as a part of who we are. We also can choose to forgive and walk in love rather than fear, which is the root of unforgiveness and bitterness.

Realizing the impact of what other people say in our own lives, we can watch the words we speak to others. Our words can heal and rewire pain or they can harm and cause pain. They can give life or death—the choice is ours.

Words are the symbolic output of the exceptional processes happening on microanatomical, epigenetic, and genetic levels in the brain. They contain power to make or break you, your loved ones, your colleagues, and your friends. Words are never just words but are a reflection of what you think about the people you speak to, including what you think about yourself.

Day 324

God's blessing on the man who endures testing! When he has passed the test, he will receive the crown of life, which God has promised to those who love him.—James 1:12

Brainy Tip: Practice really does make perfect.

Quite simply, practice makes perfect—and your brain gets healthier in the process, which in turn feeds back into your mind with positive effect. The harder and more regularly you practice taking your thoughts captive and using your thinking to your advantage, the happier and more intelligent you will be.

If you fail, pick yourself up—believe it or not, science shows we are able to do this! If you find yourself facing a challenge, persevere. You have the wisdom, strength, and power of the Holy Spirit inside you. You can live according to his glory. You are able to change your world with your thoughts. The question is not where this power is but rather how you will use it.

Day 325

*After all, God himself is the one who's at work among you,
who provides both the will and the energy to enable you to do
what pleases him. There must be no grumbling and disputing
in anything you do.—Philippians 2:13–14*

> **Brainy Tip:** Attitudes affect decisions.

Have you ever wondered why you just said that terrible thing,
or did something you know you shouldn't have done? Do you
ever wish you could go back in time and change your reaction?
Do you ever think, *What just came over me?*

Toxic moods affect our ability to think clearly and make
good decisions. Good decisions don't just happen—you pre-
pare for them by carefully checking your attitude, which is a
reflection of your character or your worldview. Healthy attitudes lead to good, healthy decisions. And, in the same way,
destructive toxic decisions can be traced back to bad attitudes.

Watch your attitude, for it has the power to affect your life.

Day 326

Stay in control of yourselves; stay awake. Your enemy, the devil, is stalking around like a roaring lion, looking for someone to devour.—1 Peter 5:8

> **Brainy Tip:** The more you focus on something negative, the more power you give to the negative.

Attention is like watering a plant. The more you water a plant, the more it grows. Likewise, the more attention you give to a thought, the more it grows in your head. If these thoughts are positive, then the water is life-giving. If these thoughts are negative, however, then the water is poisonous.

Remember, your brain is plastic—it can change and it can grow. Like positive thoughts, toxic thoughts also grow in your brain, but not in beneficial ways. Toxic thoughts upset the chemical feedback loops in your brain by putting your body into a harmful state. The growth in your brain will not be intelligent or life-enhancing. Instead, these thoughts weigh down your whole body, mind, and spirit. Your brain will grow heavy, with thick memories that release their toxic load and interfere with optimal functioning. You will lose your sense of peace and ability to think, speak, and act wisely.

Day 327

Even though I walk through the darkest valley, I fear no evil; for you are with me; your rod and your staff—they comfort me.—Psalm 23:4

Brainy Tip: In just a few days you will start to see the benefit of a renewed lifestyle.

When you set your mind to consciously take control of your thought life, you will find that it doesn't take long for the benefits to set in. Research shows that an enriched environment of thinking positive, healthy thoughts can lead to significant structural changes in the brain's cortex in only four days. Frequent and challenging (positive) learning experiences can build intelligence in a relatively short amount of time!

Renewing your mind brings health, joy, and satisfaction into your life, so push through the hard times and remind yourself that the valley you are going through is the darkness before the dawn. God has got your back; you do not have to face your problems alone or ill-equipped. You have the mind of the Messiah, so use it!

Day 328

The weapons we use for the fight, you see, are not merely human; they carry a power from God that can tear down fortresses! We tear down clever arguments and every proud notion that sets itself up against the knowledge of God.
—*2 Corinthians 10:4–5*

Brainy Tip: You control the thoughts that control your words.

The five senses are the connection between the external world and the internal world of your mind. They are the bridge between the body and your inner life, your consciousness. Information is fed into your mind constantly from your senses, shaping your thought life. In turn, the words you speak feed back into the mind, reinforcing the memory they came from. This cycle of thought can be controlled—you can choose what you want in your head, and you can choose the kind of words that come out of your mouth.

When we make negative statements, we release negative chemicals. These lead to negative memories that grow stronger and become negative strongholds that control our attitudes and lives.

What kinds of strongholds have you faced or are you facing? How did they take root in your mind? What influence do they have over your life?

Day 329

Whatever you do, do it with love.—1 Corinthians 16:14

> **Brainy Tip:** Love positively affects our physical health.

If there is one word of advice I can give anyone, it is to tune in to the power of love. Studies show clear changes in the patterns of activity of the autonomic nervous system, immune system, hormonal system, brain, and heart when you experience emotions such as appreciation, love, care, and compassion. Love is the most powerful force in the universe because God is love.

When you experience true, authentic love, your heart speeds up its communication with your mind and body through your blood flow. Life is in the blood (it is the body's transport system), and the heart is in charge of making sure the transport works. Health essentially travels from the brain to the heart in electrical signals and then through to the rest of the body! Love, in a short amount of time, can saturate the body with healthy signals and chemicals.

Day 330

Take care not to despise one of these little ones. I tell you this: in heaven, their angels are always gazing on the face of my father who lives there.—Matthew 18:10

Brainy Tip: Childhood is a particularly crucial time for the brain because neural sculpting is at its lifetime high.

Many of our abilities, tendencies, talents, and reactions are hardwired in childhood and set a mental and physical stage for adulthood. In fact, research has indicated that if children do not get enough loving touch, affection, and eye contact during the first three years of life, when their brains are organizing for independence, their emotional development can be stunted.

Of course, it isn't possible to eliminate stress on children. We cannot lock away our children to protect them from the world. However, love can help to reduce the negative effects of stress, both in childhood and in adulthood. Love is proven to be one of the most effective tools in de-stressing both children and adults!

Day 331

But the wisdom that comes from above is first holy, then peaceful, gentle, compliant, filled with mercy and good fruits, unbiased, sincere.—James 3:17

Brainy Tip: True wisdom takes time.

When you think deeply to understand, you go beyond just storing facts and answers to storing key concepts and strategies that can help you come up with your own answers. You go beyond a superficial veneer of knowledge to a deep and dynamic sense of wisdom.

Wisdom essentially means that the thoughts you have chosen to build into your mind (through intentional, deep focus) have been consolidated and stabilized sufficiently so that you have immediate access to them and can apply them to every area of your life. When this happens, you have achieved a level of expertise—*wisdom*.

You do not just "get" wisdom. You have to develop it over time by choosing to focus on positive, life-giving thoughts—thoughts of peace, gentleness, love, and mercy. You have to *learn* to think, speak, and act in wisdom.

Day 332

Blessings on the pure in heart! You will see God.—Matthew 5:8

Brainy Tip: If you listen to your heart you will learn to make decisions that bring you peace.

Your heart is not just a pump; it helps with decision-making and choices, acting like a checking station for all the emotions generated by the flow of chemicals from thoughts. Your heart is in constant communication with your brain and the rest of your body, checking the accuracy and integrity of your thought life.

As you are about to make a decision, your heart pops in with a quiet word of advice—a sense that something is right or wrong. It is well worth listening to this advice, because when you listen to your heart, it secretes the ANF (atrial natriuretic factor). ANF is a hormone produced by the heart that regulates blood pressure and can give you a feeling of peace that you are making the right decision, which in turn will promote mental and physical wellbeing.

Day 333

So take special care how you conduct yourselves. Don't be unwise, but be wise.—Ephesians 5:15

> **Brainy Tip:** You are able to mentally rehearse your actions, and that rehearsal helps you observe your own thinking and renew your mind.

Rehearsing things mentally is a great everyday example of how you can think and deeply reflect on your daily actions. Each time you do this, you change your memories and become aware of your thinking, as well as how your thinking can improve or change. You are like a surgeon who mentally rehearses each step of a complicated operation, or an athlete mentally rehearsing his or her moves before a game. As you mentally rehearse your thoughts, the newly built memory becomes increasingly stronger and begins to grow more connections to neighboring nerve cells, integrating that thought into other thought patterns. You are able to understand your thought pattern in light of your mindset, and act on it or change it to improve your mental and physical performance. This is wisdom in action.

Day 334

Bless the LORD, O my soul. O LORD my God, you are very great. You are clothed with honor and majesty, wrapped in light as with a garment.—Psalm 104:1–2

> **Brainy Tip:** Your thinking carries authority because it is customized.

Essentially, your customized thinking is your exclusive quantum state designed for *you* by God. Like a symphony orchestra, every structure in your brain has a unique role to play to make the music of your thoughts heard. There is an infinite combination of possibilities that can produce a sound that is unique each time it is played *and* heard. In fact, the experience of the previous symphony colors the current symphony, providing a new level of complexity and quality. As the warm-up of an orchestra has no identifiable tune but is still an organized process, so is the warm-up cycle of our thinking: it eventually produces a product that is beautifully whole—a magnificent symphony and a magnificent thought.

Your customized mode of thinking can never be replicated or repeated, because each experience you have had cannot be repeated. Indeed, reliving old memories or experiences adds a new layer of experience, rendering the old one as retold or reconceptualized. *Your* experience has already changed *your* thinking.

Essentially, every thought you have is a complex piece of music you have written with your choices, a piece that plays out in your brain and in your life.

Day 335

All bitterness and rage, all anger and yelling, and all blasphemy—put it all away from you, with all wickedness.
—Ephesians 4:31

> **Brainy Tip:** Toxic thinking affects your ability to handle emotions.

The amygdala, a double almond–shaped structure located in your brain, is designed to keep you emotionally alert. It steps up to protect you from any threat to your body and mind—such as danger or stress. It puts the passion behind the punch of memory formation by influencing another structure that is very important to memory formation, the hippocampus, enabling you to give more focused attention to your existing memories. The amygdala is basically designed to deal with positive love-based emotions like joy and happiness, but it doesn't work as well when you are in a negative state of mind. When you think badly, you cannot deal with your emotions wisely. You are more likely to overreact and go into a "fighting mode" if you think badly, which will harm not only you but also those around you.

Day 336

So you too must be ready! The son of man is coming at a time you don't expect.—Matthew 24:44

Brainy Tip: We need to be aware of what influences our thinking.

If we want to live the good life, we have to develop a disciplined thought life, and part of that is increasing our awareness of what we are allowing into our minds. Are we easily influenced by the external world? Or are we captives of our internal ruminations, constantly replaying negative events?

Becoming aware of all the signals that are coming into your mind from the external environment through the five senses and understanding the internal environment of your mind are incredibly important if you want to renew your mind and change the way you live your life. When you focus on developing this awareness, you start the process of bringing rogue thoughts into captivity and building new, healthy thoughts.

We must be constantly aware of the world around us and the mental world inside us. We must constantly strive to follow the example of Jesus and live a life of love and service.

Day 337

The appetite of the diligent is richly supplied.—Proverbs 13:4

Brainy Tip: We are more than capable of overcoming challenges if we persevere and change the way we think.

The best way to change, learn, and build memory meaningfully is through deliberate and disciplined practice, not mindless repetition. This includes setting deliberate, conscious goals, obtaining immediate feedback, and concentrating as much on the process as on the outcome. This will work best when you set the challenge just beyond the edge of your comfort zone. We are designed as deeply intelligent beings, and our minds and brains are created to respond to and overcome challenges.

You are made from God's perfection, but it is up to you to create your expertise in life. God gives you the blueprint, but you need to choose to make it happen. Remember, you are playing to win—don't give up.

Day 338

But if we hope for what we don't see, we wait for it eagerly—but also patiently.—Romans 8:25

Brainy Tip: Some thinking patterns take longer to change than others.

At the end of sixty-three days, you can integrate a new healthy thought into your lifestyle, into your repertoire of reactions to life. It can take anywhere from three to four twenty-one-day cycles to automatize this new healthy thought pattern and to make sure the toxic thought doesn't grow back. This process also depends on the individual, the thought pattern you are detoxing, and the healthy replacement pattern you are building. For some thoughts it might take only one twenty-one-day cycle, and for other, more toxic thought patterns, it will take more.

Be patient with yourself. Don't expect to change your mind overnight—this is impossible. Persistence is the key to successfully renewing the mind, so keep on keeping on!

Day 339

Whatever your hand finds to do, do with your might.—Ecclesiastes 9:10

> **Brainy Tip:** Renewing the mind is a lifestyle, not a one-off challenge.

Once you have started renewing your mind, don't stop! At the end of a twenty-one-day cycle of renewing the mind, the toxic thought is gone and the new healthy thought is like a tiny new plant that will need nurturing to grow—our thinking is that "nurturing." This means that if you don't practice using the new thought for another two cycles of twenty-one days, it will not be properly automatized, and it is very possible that your mind will shift back to regrowing that toxic thought and thinking, speaking, and acting according to that negative mindset.[1]

Remember, there is no instant cure for negative thinking habits.

Day 340

Yes: it's out of his fullness that we have all received, grace indeed on top of grace.—John 1:16

Brainy Tip: Thinking deeply changes the brain.

When you think deeply and are learning, many things change in the brain. For example, BDNF (brain derived neurotrophic factor) is released to consolidate the connections between neurons to enhance recall in the future. This BDNF also promotes an increase of the fatty substance called myelin, which insulates the nerves. This is a good thing, because increased myelination means faster thinking and better memory. As you start paying attention and focusing your thinking, BDNF is released, and this in turn increases attention by activating the nucleus basalis. And when the nucleus basalis is turned on, the brain becomes extremely plastic and ready to change, build, and rewire—and therefore renew.

BDNF is just another example of God's grace in our lives. No matter where we have been, no matter what we have thought, we can change. We are not in bondage to our past.

Day 341

Never stop praying.—1 Thessalonians 5:17

> **Brainy Tip:** We should never stop trying to change.

As you move into deep, focused reflection, your brain will have moments of insight accompanied by bursts of high-frequency gamma waves. These create an ideal mindset for change and learning across the brain. Neurons have their own rhythmic activity, almost like internal chatter, and changes in these fluctuations underlie how we perceive things. It is our choice to pay attention that influences this internal chatter in a positive or negative direction. You want as much of this happening as possible, because it will enhance the quality of your thinking. We need to be almost obsessive in our desire to change our thinking and renew the mind so that we can reflect God's love into the world!

Day 342

The spirit comes alongside and helps us in our weakness.
—Romans 8:26

> **Brainy Tip:** We do not have to go through life with unnecessary thoughts weighing us down.

We often go through life with unnecessary baggage—literally and figuratively. The toxic thoughts in our minds become toxic physical baggage in our brains, and because our brains are wired for love and healthy functioning, this baggage causes brain damage.

It's important to take the time to ask the Holy Spirit to show us what thoughts to change and what to focus on in our lives. Every time we feel the prompting of the Spirit, we should take that thought captive before it causes chaos in our brain and body, affecting our mental and spiritual development.

Day 343

So [we] are being changed into the same image, from glory to glory, just as you'd expect from the Lord, the spirit.
—2 Corinthians 3:18

Brainy Tip: We improve our brain function the deeper we think and the more we detox our brain.

Understanding is a complex process that cannot be computed or mechanized; it is unique to each of us. After an appropriate amount of preparation, such as reading, thinking, talking, or listening, your unique perceptions express themselves through your thoughts, words, and actions, which are not measurable or restricted to a specific area in your brain that is common to all humans. The more you do this, the more your mind is in action and the more you are increasing your brain health and wisdom—you "are being changed into the same image [of Jesus], from glory to glory."

Day 344

In the beginning was the Word. The Word was close beside God, and the Word was God.—John 1:1

> **Brainy Tip:** With our thinking, feeling, and choosing, we impact the regulatory language of our DNA and structural change occurs in the brain.

As mentioned so many times already, we need to remember what it means to be made in the image of a powerful God who brought the earth into existence with his *thoughts and words* (Gen. 1:3, 6, 9; 1 John 1:1), and that we in turn have this power of words and language invested in us (Eccles. 7:29; 2 Tim. 1:7)! In John 1:1, "Word" in Greek is *logos*, or intelligibility, reason, or intelligence, so when we operate in our image-bearing nature—our Perfect You—we activate this "Word" power with our thinking, feeling, and choosing, and we impact the regulatory language of our DNA. In turn, healthy thinking, which I call Perfect You thinking, activates our DNA and structural change occurs in the brain: this is intelligence and wisdom.

Logically, the converse is also true. Stepping out of our Perfect You–type thinking still activates the regulatory language of our DNA, but because the signal of the words is toxic, going against our image-bearing nature, this affects how proteins actually fold. A toxic thought, which is the opposite of wisdom, is born. This has a disruptive and damaging effect in the brain.

Day 345

You'll have trouble in the world. But cheer up! I have defeated the world!—John 16:33

Brainy Tip: If you put your mind to it, you can achieve what God says you can achieve.

What I saw in many of the people I worked with over the years was a mindset that *chose* to change and excel. Many of my patients *chose* not to allow their difficult life experiences to block them from succeeding. They *chose* to change. They *chose* not to succumb to the pressure nor get stuck in a neutral position and settle for the status quo.

To detox your thought life, you need to remember it's your thinking that will actually change your brain. You need to wire in positive thought networks that can fill you with the power to get back on track. You have to *choose* to have a controlled thought life, which is the foundation of happiness and health.

Day 346

Well then: you must be perfect, just as your heavenly father is perfect.—Matthew 5:48

Brainy Tip: The more we think well, the more we reflect God's image of love into the world.

The hardest part about achieving peak happiness, thinking, and health is remembering that we *can* choose them. Achieving them is not accomplished by putting on a brave or happy face; nor are they attained by adopting an ostrich mentality and pretending that problems don't exist, or that everything will always be great. The way to find this state is by harnessing the neuroplasticity God has designed in our brains and choosing to rewire—or renew—our mind. This is a lifestyle that will bring us ever closer in alignment to our original design of goodness, of being made in God's image.

Day 347

The one sown among thorns is the one who hears the word, but the world's worries and the seduction of wealth choke the word and it doesn't bear fruit.—Matthew 13:22

Brainy Tip: Don't let the world tell you who you should be or how you should think.

If you cannot be happy now, you will not be happy tomorrow. Satisfaction is the precursor to happiness, and satisfaction with your life comes from within. What is the state of your mind?

We can actively choose happiness rather than letting our external and internal world of wired-in and learned thoughts, or our biology, define happiness for us. Remember, we need to wire in positive thought networks that can fill us with the power to get back on track. Who we are at our core is where true and lasting happiness lies, but this is so often blocked by who we have become, squeezed and stretched into what the world tells us we should be.

What is blocking your path to happiness and success?

Day 348

People whose lives are determined by human flesh focus their minds on matters to do with the flesh, but people whose lives are determined by the spirit focus their minds on matters to do with the spirit. Focus the mind on the flesh, and you'll die; but focus it on the spirit, and you'll have life, and peace.—Romans 8:5–6

> **Brainy Tip:** We can get rid of toxic thoughts—we are neuro-plasticians!

Evidence of the power of the mind is all around us, in stories of our own lives and those "overcoming the odds" narratives we love to hear about. In fact, we as humans have an endless fascination with how we can use our minds to change our reality. God has designed us to be victors over the flesh and conquer it, but there is a catch—conquering the flesh only has sustainability in the love of Jesus.

The property of our brains that allows them to change is called neuroplasticity. We are actually neuroplasticians, performing brain surgery at the nano, even the quantum, scale.

Our minds are truly incredible!

Day 349

I pray that the God of King Jesus our Lord, the father of glory, would give you, in your spirit, the gift of being wise, of seeing things people can't normally see, because you are coming to know him and to have the eyes of your inmost self opened to God's light. Then you will know exactly what the hope is that goes with God's call; you will know the wealth of the glory of his inheritance in his holy people.
—Ephesians 1:17–18

Brainy Tip: Your thoughts form the basis of your worldview.

Think of your mind as a filter. The nonconscious, metacognitive mind is filled with the thoughts you have been building since you were born, and they form the perceptual base from which you see life—they filter and shape all your future thoughts, words, and actions. They are the foundation of your worldview. Whatever you have focused on the most and built deep into your mind colors the way you live your life.

What have you planted into your nonconscious mind? What are the thoughts that keep you up at night? What drives the way you think, speak, and act? How healthy is your thought life? What does your filter look like?

Day 350

And you shall love the Lord your God with all your heart, and with all your soul, and with all your understanding, and with all your strength.—Mark 12:30

Brainy Tip: Your inner life is shaped by what you choose to think about.

Automatization applies to everything in your life, because everything you do and say is first a thought. This means nothing happens until you first build the thought, which is like the roots of a tree beneath the ground. The thought produces words, actions, behavior, and so on, which can be compared to the branches, leaves, flowers, and fruit you see above the ground. The roots under the ground are like the nonconscious metacognitive mind that nourishes and supports the tree, keeping it alive twenty-four hours a day. The nonconscious metacognitive mind forms the core of your inner life, or your "soul."

Day 351

The fear of the LORD is hatred of evil. Pride and arrogance and the way of evil and perverted speech I hate.—Proverbs 8:13

> **Brainy Tip:** If we act against our wired-for-love design, we cause chaos in our brains and bodies.

When we distort love and truth, we wire this perversion into our brains and, in a sense, create brain damage. This is not an exaggeration, because our brains are wired for love, not fear, and therefore all the circuits—neurochemical, neurophysiological, neurobiological, electromagnetic, and quantum— are geared up for healthy, not toxic, thinking. If we allow ourselves to think, speak, and act in toxic fear, it creates chaos and havoc in our brains.

When we operate outside of our Perfect You, our customized, love-based way of thinking, we go into the "fear zone" and experience toxic stress. Out of this fear flows hate, anger, bitterness, rage, irritation, unforgiveness, unkindness, worry, self-pity, envy, jealousy, obsession, cynicism, and all types of "perverted speech." Research showing that love mindsets are the norm and fear mindsets are learned is revolutionary for scientists, but not new if you look at Scripture.

Day 352

When you search for me, you will find me; if you seek me with all your heart.—Jeremiah 29:13

> **Brainy Tip:** Positive plasticity produces positive behavior, and negative plasticity produces negative behavior.

Current neuroscientific and quantum physics research indicates that our thoughts change our brains on a daily, moment-by-moment basis. These changes are directed by where we choose to focus our attention. Repeated attention and effort will make learning take place. This process is called the Quantum Zeno Effect (QZE) in quantum physics. This goes hand in hand with what neuroscience literature has coined as "self-directed neuroplasticity." This is a general description of the principle that deep thinking continually changes brain structure and function. This plastic ability of the brain to change in a positive or negative direction, depending on our state of mind, is called the plastic paradox. Positive QZE produces positive behavior, and negative QZE produces negative behavior.

It is up to us to choose which direction we want our minds to go. Jesus does not force us to follow his way of love—we have to choose to "find" him. We have to choose to follow him by choosing to focus on things that build up, rather than tear down, our wired-for-love design.

Day 353

"Get out of here, you satan!" replied Jesus. "The Bible says, 'Worship the Lord your God, and serve him alone!'"
—Matthew 4:10

> **Brainy Tip:** You can choose to believe the lies of the satan or the promises of God. Your choices turn these probabilities into realities.

It's through the senses that we receive the satan's lies, but—and this is important—we don't have to believe those lies. If we do believe them, we process them into physical realities (through the conscious cognitive to the nonconscious meta-cognitive) that form the substance of the nerve networks upon which we act. This means that if we listen to and believe the enemy's lies, we actually choose to process them into physical realities inside our brains. In doing so, we create the evil and act upon it. We do not have to believe the satan's lies. We collapse our probabilities into actualities.

As human beings with free will, we create chaos when we collapse negative, toxic probabilities into actualities through our choices. God has given us the power to create good or evil with our choices. Once we are aware of these very real consequences, we will hopefully be more cautious when it comes to using our powerful minds.

Day 354

When I am afraid, I put my trust in you. In God, whose word I praise, in God I trust; I am not afraid; what can flesh do to me?—Psalm 56:3–4

Brainy Tip: We do not have to live our lives afraid and defeated.

Although we feel the pull of the sensory information coming into our minds, we don't have to be controlled by the events and circumstances of the world. We need to keep reminding ourselves that we cannot control life's events and circumstances—but we can control our reactions to them.

We don't have to just react to what happens to us or accept what comes our way without fighting back with our minds and our choices. We can take the time to slow down and think about how we should react—about how we can overcome whatever life throws our way. After all, giving up is a choice. If we build healthy, encouraging, and determined thought patterns into our minds, we can change the way we respond to the circumstances of life, thereby changing the way we live our life. We do not have to live our lives as if we have already been defeated.

Day 355

Some seed fell on rocky soil, where it didn't have much earth.
It sprang up at once because it didn't have depth of soil. But
when the sun was high it got scorched, and it withered because
it didn't have any root.—Matthew 13:5–6

Brainy Tip: If you stop working on something daily, the memory
will denature and die.

You can't just apply a thought once and think change has
happened. It takes repeated work to build healthy thinking
patterns. Each day something is happening to the thought in
your nonconscious mind. If you give up at day four or five,
which people often do, then the consequence will be that
the memory denatures—which means it dies and becomes
heat energy. Simply put, you forget; all the effort you put into
changing your thinking literally becomes "hot air." Giving
up puts you two steps behind in life.

Day 356

God's people should make petitions, prayers, intercessions, and thanksgivings on behalf of all people—on behalf of kings, and all who hold high office, so that we may lead a tranquil and peaceful life, in all godliness and holiness.
—1 Timothy 2:1–2

Brainy Tip: Prayer reflects the entangled nature of the universe.

The law of entanglement in quantum physics states that relationship is the defining characteristic of everything in space and time. Because of the pervasive nature of the entanglement of atomic particles, relationship is independent of distance and requires no physical link. Everything and everyone is linked, and we all affect each other.

Quantum theory calls entanglement bizarre behavior for particles, such as two entangled particles behaving as one even when far apart. Physicists call such behavior nonlocal, which means that it is physically impossible to know the position and the momentum of a particle at the same time. Another way of saying this is that there is no space-time dimension.

We know God operates outside of the space-time dimension. And we know prayer does too. There are many stories of people praying for each other on different sides of the planet and experiencing the effect of that prayer. In fact, there are many documented studies on the impact of prayer in the world of neuroscience, in addition to the millions of testimonies from people around the world. The power of prayer highlights the power of entanglement: what we think and what we hope for can affect not only us but the whole world.

Day 357

Celebrate with those who are celebrating; mourn with the mourners. Come to the same mind with one another.
—Romans 12:15–16

Brainy Tip: The brain reflects the entangled nature of the universe.

We are entangled in each other's lives, and this entanglement is reflected in the structure of the brain. We have mirror neurons that fire up as we watch someone else laugh or cry or drink a cup of coffee. This means we literally fire up activity in the brain without actually using our five senses through the normal sensory-cognitive cycle!

Empathy is the wonderful God-given ability to identify with, and vicariously understand, the internal experiences of another person. It makes communication more genuine and valuable. When we empathize, many different regions of the brain collaborate in addition to the tiny little miracles, the mirror-neurons. We have been hardwired to experience powerful compassion and love for others.

Day 358

Never repay anyone evil for evil; think through what will seem good to everyone who is watching. If it's possible, as far as you can, live at peace with all people.—Romans 12:17–18

Brainy Tip: What we think, say, and do has the power to affect the lives of people everywhere.

We are all part of God, so the law of entanglement is not surprising. Your intentions, your prayers, your words toward others all will have impact because of this law. In fact, we are so entangled that our intentions alter not only our own DNA but the DNA of others as well. So watch what you say, think, and feel, because you never know the full impact you have on others.

Day 359

Then our mouth was filled with laughter, and our tongue with shouts of joy; then it was said among the nations, "The LORD has done great things for them." The LORD has done great things for us, and we rejoiced.—Psalm 126:2–3

> **Brainy Tip:** Don't take life too seriously; it is not good for your health!

Sometimes we get so caught up in the cycle of toxic thoughts and emotions and words and choices that we forget who we are—our true selves—and we seem to operate like automatons, just doing what we are supposed to do and barely surviving. We can become too serious about life!

Having fun will detox your mind, improving your health and making you clever to boot because your unique way of thinking is neurologically developed when you have fun. Having fun is one of the most powerful antidotes to toxic stress you will ever find. And it's free! It's a tremendous resource God has built into your brain to bring perspective into your life, help surmount problems, add sizzle to your relationships, and make you feel good.

I love having fun with my children. They do the craziest things and say the funniest things that make me laugh. I love going for walks with them and the dogs and hearing their stories. I love sitting with them and making up silly songs and voices and anything that makes us laugh. If we allowed our schedules to take over our lives, we never would have these important, life-giving moments.

Day 360

Brainy Tip: Our reactions affect our mental and physical health.

Our bodies react to both physical attacks and mental alarm in a similar fashion by a process called inflammation. Inflammation, if short-lived, is beneficial. However, if it is prolonged it can physically damage the brain and body.

Among the substances first released in the inflammatory process is the appropriately named C-reactive protein, a five-part protein produced in the liver. A number of researchers have found that worrying about a past stressful event, known as toxic rumination, is associated with persistently high levels of C-reactive protein in the blood, indicating chronic inflammation in the body, which is associated with mental and physical disorders.

We cannot control our circumstances; however, we can control our reactions to those circumstances. And it seems our reactions can be measured by C-reactive protein. If we react the wrong way, we can damage our brains and bodies. If we react to our circumstances in the right way, we can bring health and healing to our brains and bodies.

Day 361

Happy are those who find wisdom, and those who get understanding, for her income is better than silver, and her revenue better than gold. She is more precious than jewels, and nothing you desire can compare with her. Long life is in her right hand; in her left hand are riches and honor. Her ways are ways of pleasantness, and all her paths are peace. She is a tree of life to those who lay hold of her; those who hold her fast are called happy.—Proverbs 3:13–18

Brainy Tip: No matter where we are in our lives, we can develop our wisdom and use our minds to change the way we think, thereby changing the way we live.

When you adopt a lifestyle of intense mental focus, you quite literally "switch on" neuroplasticity, the marvelous ability of the brain to grow branches and unending scaffolds of networks to increase your wisdom. Strategic approaches to thinking will create new neural pathways and strengthen existing ones for as long as you live!

Indeed, it does not matter how sick or mentally challenged we may feel, we still have the ability to choose our thoughts and feelings and determine the direction of our lives. God has equipped each of us with all the genetic material and epigenetic ability we need to deal optimally with the challenges that come our way.

Day 362

The righteousness of the righteous shall be his own, and the wickedness of the wicked shall be his own.—Ezekiel 18:20

Brainy Tip: We have to take responsibility for our thought life.

What we think influences every aspect of who we are and how we feel physically. We cannot escape the consequences of our thinking—we have to take responsibility for the way we choose to live our lives. Our state of mind (our thought life) is quite literally determining our mental and physical health.

What does your current state of mind say about your health, mentally and physically? Think of the ways in which your thinking has impacted your life. Think of specific situations where your thinking has helped you or hindered you.

Day 363

He went on through the whole of Galilee, teaching in their synagogues and proclaiming the good news of the kingdom, healing every disease and every illness among the people.
—Matthew 4:23

Brainy Tip: Love has the power to heal.

Because of the spiritual, emotional, and chemical bond between people, we have the power to build each other up or tear each other down. This causes real structural change in our brains in a positive or negative direction—it's up to us.

If we treat each other with love, we can actually alleviate mental and physical pain! The areas of the brain activated by intense love are the same areas that drugs use to reduce pain. So do not resist feeling and expressing love for others, because there are tremendous physical benefits when you do.

It is no wonder Jesus performed so many miracles! His words and actions underscore the power of true love. Love can literally heal you and those around you.

Day 364

*For I, the L*ORD *your God, hold your right hand; it is I who say to you, "Do not fear, I will help you."*—Isaiah 41:13

Brainy Tip: Don't waste time worrying about things you cannot change.

Life throws things at us that seem to fill our brains with toxic thoughts, and they seem so hard to control. We all have experienced this helplessness. I have had many experiences that I would have preferred not to have had, and I am sure you have as well. In hindsight, I can always see God was working behind the scenes, and there is value in the lessons I have learned. But I have also seen on every occasion how, when I indulged in self-pity or worry, the fruit turned bad—I felt my thoughts were draining the life out of me. I knew I had to bring those thoughts into captivity, repent (that is, change my mind), and forgive so peace and joy would flood my being again, freeing me to be the person God created me to be.

Have you ever found yourself going to sleep thinking about a situation and then waking up thinking about the situation? Has your head ever been so filled with toxic details that it felt like you had to shake it to make room for something else? Have you ever had toxic thoughts consuming your every moment and coloring your attitude to everything?

These toxic thoughts do nothing but harm your peace and block your ability to think clearly, but the good news is that you can get rid of them by renewing your mind! Thoughts are active: they grow and change according to your choices—where you choose to direct your attention.

Day 365

Don't lose your enthusiasm for behaving properly. You'll bring in the harvest at the proper time, if you don't become weary.—Galatians 6:9

Brainy Tip: True change takes time.

Nothing worthwhile happens in an instant. We can turn dreams into realities, but we first have to realize that it takes longer than the average one-second lifespan of a Twitter post to make a change. Never give up or "lose your enthusiasm" for improving the way you live your life. I understand that in many ways the technological age has brought with it a desire to see things, including change and success, as instantaneous. Yet there is no quick fix to success or happiness in school, work, and life. Trying to make things happen fast and then giving up when they do not happen at the speed you have become accustomed to or expected is unhealthy. It can cause you anguish and put your brain and body into toxic stress, making you "weary" and affecting your ability to truly be a light in the world.

Epilogue

Congratulations! Over the past year you have begun the process of choosing to renew your mind by thinking, asking, and discussing the relationship between your mind and God's plan for your life. But remember, this process is about creating a renewed *lifestyle*, not merely completing a book.

You have been thinking deeply, and thinking deeply is essentially cardio for the brain! In fact, it's my favorite kind of exercise. Thinking deeply is incredibly beneficial for brain and mind health because it allows our minds to develop and reach their full potential, laying the foundation for long-term mind renewal.

And although changing the way you think, speak, and act may sound daunting, once you have developed a pattern of renewing your mind, it becomes easier to do—almost like second nature! When you change your thinking, you can change your life, which will enable you to offer yourself as a living sacrifice—body, mind, and spirit—every day for the rest of your days! You will be able to bring heaven to earth through your thoughts, words, and actions. You will be able to say, in all honesty, that the "kingdom of heaven is at hand."

Remember, you are a light on a hill. Don't hide what you have to give under a basket of bad thinking habits. You have the mind, and the power, of the Messiah.

Notes

Introduction

1. N. T. Wright, *Scripture and the Authority of God: How to Read the Bible Today* (New York: Harper-One, 2013), 1–60; Rob Bell, *What Is the Bible? How an Ancient Library of Poems, Letters, and Stories Can Transform the Way You Think and Feel about Everything* (San Francisco: HarperOne, 2017), 4–6, 87–93, 121–24, 151–74.

2. Ibid.

3. Thomas O'Loughlin, "The People of the Book," *The Furrow* 62, no. 4 (2011): 209–12.

4. J. C. Polkinghorne, *Quantum Physics and Theology: An Unexpected Kinship* (New Haven: Yale University Press, 2007), 109–10.

5. Ibid.

6. Caroline Leaf, *Switch On Your Brain: The Key to Peak Happiness, Thinking, and Health* (Grand Rapids: Baker, 2015), 103–22.

7. Ibid.

8. Bell, *What Is the Bible?* 4–6, 87–93, 121–24, 151–74.

9. Ibid; O'Loughlin, "The People of the Book," 209–12.

10. Bell, *What Is the Bible?* 4–6, 87–93, 121–24, 151–74.

11. Alister E. McGrath, *Surprised by Meaning: Science, Faith, and How We Make Sense of Things* (Louisville: Westminster John Knox, 2011), 1–14.

12. O'Loughlin, "The People of the Book," 209–12.

13. Bell, *What Is the Bible?* 4–6, 87–93, 121–24, 151–74.

14. N. T. Wright, *Paul and the Faithfulness of God* (Minneapolis: Fortress Press, 2013), 567.

Day 11

1. Tremper Longman III, *Proverbs* (Grand Rapids: Baker Academic, 2006), 420.

Day 23

1. N. T. Wright, *The Climax of the Covenant: Christ and the Law in Pauline Theology* (Minneapolis: Fortress Press, 1992), 185.

Day 27

1. N. T. Wright, *Lent for Everyone: A Daily Devotional, Matthew Year A* (Louisville: Westminster John Knox, 2013), 13.

Day 28

1. J. Richard Fountain, *Eschatological Relationships and Jesus in Ben F.*

Meyer, N. T. Wright, and Progressive Dispensationalism (Eugene, OR: Wipf & Stock, 2016), 131.

2. Andrew T. Lincoln, *Paradise Now and Not Yet: Studies in the Role of the Heavenly Dimension in Paul's Thought with Special Reference to His Eschatology* (Cambridge: Cambridge University Press, 2004), 1–8.

Day 29

1. Roger Penrose, *The Emperor's New Mind: Concerning Computers, Minds, and the Laws of Physics* (London: Oxford University Press, 1999).

Day 32

1. Mike Bird, "N. T. Wright: The Church Continues the Revolution Jesus Started," *Christianity Today*, October 2016, http://www.christianitytoday.com/ct/2016/october-web-only/n-t-wright-jesus-death-does-more-than-just-get-us-into-heav.html.

Day 36

1. J. Richard Middleton, *A New Heaven and a New Earth: Reclaiming Biblical Eschatology* (Grand Rapids: Baker Academic, 2014), 129–76.

Day 41

1. Henry Stapp, "Minds and Values in the Quantum Universe," in *Information and the Nature of Reality from Physics to Metaphysics*, ed. P. C. W. Davies and Niels Henrick Gregersen (Cambridge, UK: Cambridge University Press, 2014), 157.

Day 58

1. James K. A. Smith, *You Are What You Love: The Spiritual Power of Habit* (Grand Rapids: Brazos, 2016), 111.

Day 63

1. Wright, *Paul and the Faithfulness of God*, 377.

Day 64

1. N. T. Wright and Richard B. Hays, "Evening Conversation with N. T. Wright and Richard Hays (February 24, 2016)," Youtube video, 1:33:45, uploaded by The Trinity Forum, May 26, 2016, https://www.youtube.com/watch?v=w6XakC2ZjsU&index=52&list=WL.

Day 92

1. Michael Gelb and Sarah Miller Caldicott, *Innovate Like Edison: The Five-Step System for Breakthrough Business Success* (New York: Plume, 2008), 88–90.

Day 102

1. Shawn Achor, *The Happiness Advantage: The Seven Principles of Positive Psychology that Fuel Success and Performance at Work* (New York: Random House, 2011).

Day 148

1. Leaf, *Switch On Your Brain*; www.21daybraindetox.com.

2. Caroline Leaf, *The Perfect You* (Grand Rapids: Baker, 2017).

Day 159

1. Richard Swinburne, *Mind, Brain and Free Will* (London: Oxford University Press, 2013).

Day 175

1. Leaf, *Switch On Your Brain*; Leaf, *The Perfect You*; Caroline Leaf, *Think, Learn, Succeed* (Grand Rapids: Baker, 2018).

Day 189

1. Leaf, *Think, Learn, Succeed*.

Day 223

1. John H. Walton, *The Lost World of Genesis One: Ancient Cosmology and the Origins Debate* (Downers Grove, IL: InterVarsity, 2010), 72–77.

Day 230

1. Walton, *Lost World of Genesis One*, 72–77.

Day 276

1. Dan Buettner, *The Blue Zone: Lessons for Living Longer from the People Who've Lived the Longest* (Washington, DC: National Geographic, 2008), 1–22.

Day 315

1. "Religion and the Quantum World—Professor Keith Ward," Vimeo video, 50:06, uploaded by Gresham College on April 11, 2012, https://vimeo.com/40154090, run time 18:00–18:25.

Day 339

1. Leaf, *Switch On Your Brain*; www.21daybraindetox.com.

Dr. Caroline Leaf is the author of *Switch On Your Brain*, *Think and Eat Yourself Smart*, and *The Perfect You*, among many other books and journal articles. Since 1981, she has researched the science of thought and the mind-brain connection as it relates to thinking, learning, renewing the mind, gifting, and potential. Dr. Leaf practiced clinically for twenty-five years and is an international and national conference speaker on topics relating to optimal brain performance such as learning, mindful thinking, stress, toxic thoughts, male/female brain differences, mindful eating, and much more. She is frequently interviewed on TV stations around the globe, has published many books and scientific journal articles, and has her own TV show, *The Dr. Leaf Show*. She and her husband, Mac, live with their four children in Dallas and Los Angeles.

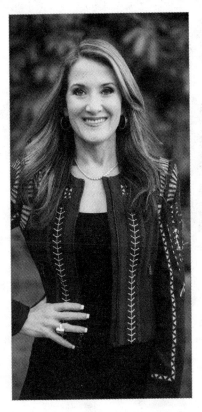

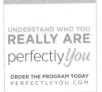

Discover the Keys to Peak
HAPPINESS, THINKING,
AND HEALTH

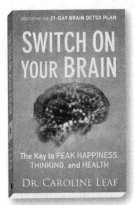

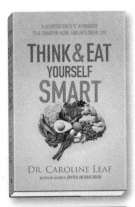

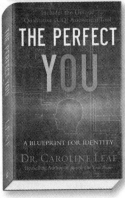

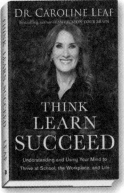